NATIONAL
ACADEMIES

Sciences
Engineering
Medicine

The Food Forum 30th Anniversary

Anna Nicholson, *Rapporteur*

Food Forum

Food and Nutrition Board

Health and Medicine Division

Proceedings of a Symposium

NATIONAL ACADEMIES PRESS 500 Fifth Street, NW Washington, DC 20001

This activity was supported by contracts between the National Academy of Sciences and National Institutes of Health (HHSN263201800029I/ 75N98023F00028), the U.S. Department of Agriculture (59-8040-3-001 and 123A9423P0005), and the U.S. Food and Drug Administration (75F40120C00192), with additional support from the American Heart Association; American Society for Nutrition; Cargill, Inc.; The Coca-Cola Company; Conagra Brands; Center for Science in the Public Interest; Danone North America; General Mills, Inc.; Institute of Food Technologists; Mars, Inc.; Mondelēz International; National Council on Aging; and Ocean Spray Cranberries, Inc. Any opinions, findings, conclusions, or recommendations expressed in this publication do not necessarily reflect the views of any organization or agency that provided support for the project.

International Standard Book Number-13: 978-0-309-71920-9
International Standard Book Number-10: 0-309-71920-8
Digital Object Identifier: https://doi.org/10.17226/27771

This publication is available from the National Academies Press, 500 Fifth Street, NW, Keck 360, Washington, DC 20001; (800) 624-6242; http://www.nap.edu.

Printed in the United States of America.

Suggested citation: National Academies of Sciences, Engineering, and Medicine. 2024. *The Food Forum 30th anniversary: Proceedings of a symposium.* Washington, DC: National Academies Press. https://doi.org/10.17226/27771.

PLANNING COMMITTEE FOR FOOD FORUM
30TH ANNIVERSARY SYMPOSIUM

ERIC A. DECKER (*Chair*), Professor, Department of Food Science, University of Massachusetts Amherst

DOUGLAS BALENTINE, Senior Science Advisor, International Nutrition Policy, Center for Food Safety and Applied Nutrition, U.S. Food and Drug Administration

CHRISTINA KHOO, Director, Emerging Science, Nutrition and Regulatory Affairs, Ocean Spray Cranberries, Inc.

MEGAN NECHANICKY, Nutrition Manager, North America Retail and Global Health & Wellness, General Mills, Inc.

SHARON A. ROSS, Program Director, Nutrition Science Research Group, Division of Cancer Prevention, National Cancer Institute, National Institutes of Health

SYLVIA B. ROWE, President, SR Strategy, LLC

PAMELA STARKE-REED, Deputy Administrator, Nutrition, Food Safety, and Quality, Agricultural Research Service, U.S. Department of Agriculture

MARY T. STORY, Professor, Global Health and Family Medicine and Community Health, Duke University

PATRICK J. STOVER, Professor, Director, Institute for Advancing Health Through Agriculture, Texas A&M University

FOOD FORUM (AS OF NOVEMBER 2023)

ERIC A. DECKER (*Chair*), University of Massachusetts Amherst
RODOLPHE BARRANGOU, North Carolina State University, Raleigh
WENDY ATTAYA BOLAND, Kogod School of Business, American
   University, Washington, DC
CINDY DAVIS, Agricultural Research Service, U.S. Department of
   Agriculture, Beltsville, Maryland
DENISE R. EBLEN, Food Safety and Inspection Service, U.S. Department
   of Agriculture, Washington, DC
EMILY DIMIERO, Federal Government Relations, Cargill, Washington, DC
NAOMI K. FUKAGAWA, Agricultural Research Service, U.S. Department
   of Agriculture, Beltsville, Maryland
JAIME J. GAHCHE, Office of Dietary Supplements, National Institutes
   of Health, Bethesda, Maryland
CUTBERTO GARZA, Cornell University, Ithaca, New York
STEPHANIE K. GOODWIN, Danone North America, Washington, DC
M. R. C. GREENWOOD, University of California, Davis
MARTIN HAHN, Hogan Lovells, Washington, DC
BRYAN HITCHCOCK, Institute of Food Technologists, Chicago, Illinois
TERRY T-K HUANG, City University of New York School of Public
   Health and Health Policy, New York City
EVA HURT, The Coca-Cola Company, Atlanta, Georgia
RENÉE S. JOHNSON, Congressional Research Service, Library of
   Congress, Washington, DC
CHRISTINA KHOO, Ocean Spray Cranberries, Inc., Lakeville,
   Massachusetts
CASEY LEWIS, Director, Nutrition and Regulatory Affairs, Clif Bar,
   Mondelēz International
ALICE H. LICHTENSTEIN, Tufts University, Boston, Massachusetts
PETER LURIE, Center for Science in the Public Interest, Washington, DC
MEGAN NECHANICKY, General Mills, Inc., Golden Valley, Minnesota
RONI NEFF, Johns Hopkins University, Baltimore, Maryland
SAM R. NUGEN, Cornell University, Ithaca, New York
SARAH OHLHORST, American Society for Nutrition, Rockville,
   Maryland
HALEY F. OLIVER, Purdue University, West Lafayette, Indiana
DONALD A. PRATER, Center for Food Safety and Nutrition, U.S. Food
   and Drug Administration, College Park, Maryland
JILL REEDY, Division of Cancer Prevention, National Cancer Institute,
   National Institutes of Health, Bethesda, Maryland
KRISTIN REIMERS, Conagra Brands, Omaha, Nebraska

Reviewers

This proceedings of a symposium was reviewed in draft form by individuals chosen for their diverse perspectives and technical expertise. The purpose of this independent review is to provide candid and critical comments that will assist the National Academies of Sciences, Engineering, and Medicine in making each published proceedings as sound as possible and to ensure that it meets the institutional standards for quality, objectivity, evidence, and responsiveness to the charge. The review comments and draft manuscript remain confidential to protect the integrity of the process.

We thank the following individuals for their review of this proceedings:

DOUGLAS BALENTINE, U.S. Food and Drug Administration
ALISON G. M. BROWN, National Institutes of Health
PATRICK J. STOVER, Texas A&M University

Although the reviewers listed above provided many constructive comments and suggestions, they were not asked to endorse the content of the proceedings, nor did they see the final draft before its release. The review of this proceedings was overseen by **CHERYL A. ANDERSON,** University of California, San Diego. She was responsible for making certain that an independent examination of this proceedings was carried out in accordance with standards of the National Academies and that all review comments were carefully considered. Responsibility for the final content rests entirely with the rapporteur and the National Academies.

Contents

Acronyms and Abbreviations

AI	artificial intelligence
BVG	Branch Venture Group
COP	Conference of Parties
Danone NA	Danone North America
DEI	diversity, equity, and inclusion
E. coli	*Escherichia coli*
FDA	U.S. Food and Drug Administration
FSMA	Food Safety Modernization Act
FSVP	Foreign Supplier Verification Program
GLP-1	glucagon-like peptide 1
GMO	genetically modified organism
HACCP	hazard analysis critical control point
IT	information technology
KPI	key performance indicator
NHS	National Health Service

PFAS   per- and polyfluoroalkyl substances

UKRI   UK Research and Innovation
USAID   U.S. Agency for International Development
USDA   U.S. Department of Agriculture

1

Introduction

The Food Forum of the National Academies of Sciences, Engineering, and Medicine (the National Academies) convened the Food Forum 30th Anniversary Symposium on November 30, 2023, to celebrate its anniversary and reflect on its contributions to developments in the field of food, nutrition, and agriculture.[1] The symposium reviewed the history of the Food Forum, its evolution, and how it has informed research, policy, and industry practice. The symposium also featured discussions on the future of food in light of challenges such as climate change and population growth, new technologies to address these challenges, how these challenges affect and are influenced by health equity issues, and how the Food Forum will continue to approach these issues proactively and through a multisectoral lens.

The true impact of the Food Forum is woven into a much larger narrative about food and nutrition science and action in the United States—specifically, increased awareness around food safety and the federal government's response to food safety threats. As national priorities in this area shifted over the years, so did the work of the forum, leading to an impressive portfolio of scientific leadership that has touched countless lives.

The symposium opened with welcoming remarks from Monica N. Feit, executive director of the National Academies' Health and Medicine Division, who acknowledged the accomplishments of the forum over the

---

[1] The symposium agenda, presentations, and other materials are available at https://www.nationalacademies.org/event/40053_11-2023_the-food-forum-30th-anniversary-symposium (accessed February 24, 2024).

past three decades. The forum addresses a broad range of issues, she said, such as nutrition, food safety, nanotechnology, sustainable agriculture, and alternative protein sources, and its work involves reacting to and informing government and industry priorities. Feit described the forum as highlighting the National Academies' convening ability, bringing together thought leaders who are passionate about the complicated food system and creating a neutral space for science-guided discussions, brainstorming, and sharing of ideas and lessons learned. Such activities are critical to moving the nation forward in a positive direction, particularly given the current challenges to civil discourse, said Feit.

Marcia McNutt, president of the National Academy of Sciences, reflected on the significance of the forum, one of the National Academies' first convening bodies, and emphasized that its three decades of activity have advanced national dialogues in food safety, precision nutrition, food system sustainability, and more. Assembling key players from the federal government, academia, the private sector, and professional organizations, the forum confronts the most challenging and pressing issues related to food and generates benefit for the nation and the world, McNutt stated.

Planning committee chair Eric A. Decker, University of Massachusetts Amherst, highlighted that over the past 30 years, more than 180 members have served in the forum, representing industry, academia, federal government, nonprofit organizations, and consumer-oriented groups. Furthermore, Decker continued, more than 350 experts have contributed their expertise on nutrition, policy, regulation, and other areas related to the food system at forum events, and more than 200 volunteers have participated in program planning. Thousands of people have participated in the events, including approximately 1,300 people registered for this symposium. Decker underscored the forum's efforts to address challenges within the highly complex food system to produce a safe and nutritious food supply, including symposia covering groundbreaking topics, such as interactions between diet and the microbiome.

During the symposium's first session, former forum chairs discussed the forum's history, role, accomplishments, and continued relevance in addressing current and emerging challenges (Chapter 2). The second session explored issues related to food safety within the contexts of regulation, manufacturing, and developing economies (Chapter 3). The third session considered the environmental effects of the food system and approaches to increasing sustainability (Chapter 4). The fourth session examined nutrition and health through the lenses of personalized nutrition, food composition, and equity considerations (Chapter 5). The fifth session presented a vision for the future of food that reflected health, environmental, and socioeconomic effects of the food system (Chapter 6). The symposium's final session featured a discussion on technological effects within the food

> **BOX 1-1**
> **Symposium Statement of Task**
>
> A planning committee of the National Academies of Sciences, Engineering, and Medicine will be appointed to organize a one-day public symposium to explore and reflect on the major developments in the field of food, nutrition, and agriculture over the past 30 years, and how the Food Forum has contributed to those developments. The symposium will review the history of the Food Forum, its evolution, and how it has informed research, policy, and industry practice. The symposium will address areas relevant to the origin and ongoing purpose of the Food Forum, including: the role of the Food Forum as a convening activity at National Academies; how approaches to and methodologies for nutrition research have changed within the field; and the impact of Food Forum publications and activities on policy and practice. The symposium will also feature discussions on the future of food in light of challenges such as climate change and population growth, new technologies to address these challenges, how these challenges affect and are influenced by health equity issues, and how the Food Forum will continue to approach these issues proactively and through a multi-sectoral lens.

system, contextual challenges, the intersection of health span and nutrition, and consumer and industry behavior change (Chapter 7). The symposium agenda, acronyms and abbreviations used in this publication, and biographical sketches of the symposium speakers and planning committee members can be found in Appendixes A, B, and C, respectively. The symposium's statement of task is in Box 1-1.[2]

---

[2] The symposium planning committee's role was limited to planning the symposium. This proceedings of a symposium was prepared by an independent rapporteur as a factual summary of what occurred at the symposium. Statements, recommendations, and opinions expressed are those of independent presenters and participants and are not necessarily endorsed or verified by the National Academies of Sciences, Engineering, and Medicine, nor should they be construed as reflecting any group consensus.

2

History of the Food Forum and Its Impact Over the Past 30 Years

The first session of the symposium featured a discussion on the Food Forum's history, role, effects within the food system, and continued relevance. The discussion included four former forum chairs: Francis F. Busta, National Center for Food Protection and Defense (now Food Protection and Defense Institute); Fergus M. Clydesdale, University of Massachusetts Amherst; Michael P. Doyle, retired director of the Center for Food Safety at the University of Georgia; and Sylvia B. Rowe, SR Strategy. The session was moderated by the current forum chair, Eric A. Decker, University of Massachusetts Amherst.

EARLY YEARS

Decker began the discussion by soliciting insights on the importance of the forum in its initial years. Clydesdale remarked that the late 1980s and early 1990s were a transitional time in food science, production, nutrition, and regulation, with consumer activism becoming increasingly important during this period. The National Academies of Sciences, Engineering, and Medicine created the forum to establish a public–private partnership capable of changing the food supply through collaboration with food producers and regulators. Convening representatives from academia, regulatory agencies, consumer policy, food production, food technology, and nutrition, the forum generates independent thinking and stimulates solutions, Clydesdale said.

Doyle noted a major disconnect in the early 1990s between the government and the food industry regarding food safety regulations and oversight.

He said the forum established a neutral setting for leaders in the food industry and in the federal government—specifically, the U.S. Food and Drug Administration (FDA) and the U.S. Department of Agriculture (USDA)—to address these issues collaboratively.

CHAIR TENURE HIGHLIGHTS

Decker invited each former chair to share key events during their respective tenures leading the forum.

Rowe, who served as chair from 2015 to 2021, underscored the challenges that the COVID-19 pandemic posed to the forum. Personal relationships and interactions are fundamental to the success of the forum's role as a convening body, she said. Therefore, the forum had to determine how to continue its interactions and adapt its programming to virtual platforms, given the pandemic-related restrictions on travel and gathering. Additionally, Rowe stated, the pandemic accelerated and amplified numerous issues fundamental both to public dialogue and to groups participating in the forum. Such issues included food and nutrition security, obesity, the rise in noncommunicable diseases, and climate change, all of which involve social justice considerations. She added that, as issues facing the forum evolved and broadened, the forum diversified by including consumer groups as well as scientific and professional societies to maximize the knowledge and experience within the group.

Busta, the forum's chair from 2011 to 2014, emphasized the key role of interaction in forum activities, which enables participants to discuss issues not typically addressed in open forums. Workshops during his tenure focused on topics including public–private partnerships; the influence of food on the human microbiome and on health; sustainable diets; and the relationships among the brain, the digestive system, and eating behavior. He noted that these workshops preceded much of the research activity and government regulations that would later address these issues.

Doyle, forum chair from 2003 to 2011, noted the role of the forum on FDA regulation regarding hazard analysis critical control points (HACCPs). When the forum was initiated, FDA required the food industry to apply an HACCP program to every food produced. During a meeting early in the forum's history, Doyle stated, discussion regarding this requirement featured a debate between representatives from the food industry and FDA. A food company executive stressed that some foods, such as saltine crackers, do not pose hazards and thus do not require HACCP plans. Doyle said that this debate led FDA to conduct a hazard analysis on all foods and adjust HACCP rules to require plans only on foods that pose a hazard.

Clydesdale, forum chair from 1996 to 2002, highlighted the value that participants from FDA and USDA bring to the forum. He remarked that spirited debate at forum meetings has stimulated actions such as FDA's sponsorship of a keystone committee that finalized regulations on health claims.

ROLE IN THE FIELD

Decker asked the participants to discuss the role of the forum in policy, regulation, research, and scientific communications. Doyle reiterated that the shift in HACCP rule application was catalyzed by forum discussions. Clydesdale remarked on the powerful role of the forum in forging connections across science, production, regulation, research, communications, and policy to best meet the needs of consumers. He noted that the forum played a role in structure/function claims, which in turn led to front-of-package labeling that makes helpful information more accessible to consumers. Busta underscored that the forum does not make recommendations for regulations, but interactions at forum events have played a role in regulation. He said the forum offers academics a rare opportunity to discuss regulations, healthy foods, and healthy diets with representatives from industry and government, thereby providing academics an opportunity to inform policy. Rowe commented that the academic community has responded to research needs and gaps identified in forum dialogues. She added that in each topic of focus, the forum considers issues of equity, communications, and data—facets that are sometimes lost in broader discussions.

ROLE IN THE FUTURE

Regarding the role that the forum may play in the future, Busta emphasized that the current digital age minimizes personal, direct interactions; within this context, the forum is essential in providing opportunities for interaction, connection, problem-solving, idea sharing, and exposure to topics that participants may not have considered. Doyle remarked on the forum's focus on food safety, nutrition, and related cutting-edge issues. For instance, he said, food safety concerns with fresh produce have yet to be fully addressed. The forum provides a unique, neutral setting in which leaders from regulatory agencies and academia can collaborate to address such issues. Rowe stated her optimism about the future of the forum, citing the need for public–private partnerships and highlighting the opportunities the forum provides. She commended the forum's staff, whom she described as "committed and talented," for enabling the interaction of forum members. Rowe continued, these transdisciplinary interactions—conducted in a neutral, safe environment—address the pressing need to collapse silos within the food system space. Clydesdale noted current partisanship within society and the need for cooperation to solve problems.

The forum provides opportunities for collaborative problem-solving within the milieu of partisanship, he observed. Clydesdale noted burgeoning issues that will require legislation, including food as medicine, artificial intelligence and precision nutrition, local farm production to temper climate change, gene editing to create produce that can withstand altered climates, and safe utilization of waste.

Decker concluded the discussion by acknowledging Richard L. Hall, who served as the first forum chair from 1992 to 1996 and played an instrumental role in creating a strong foundation for the forum's three decades of activity. Hall passed away in 2019 at the age of 96.

3

Food Safety

The second session of the symposium featured three presentations and a discussion on food safety developments and challenges from a regulatory perspective and a manufacturing perspective, and within the context of developing economies. The session was moderated by Sam R. Nugen, Cornell University.

REGULATORY PERSPECTIVE

Susan T. Mayne, former director of the Center for Food Safety and Applied Nutrition at the U.S. Food and Drug Administration (FDA), provided a regulatory perspective on food safety progress and considerations for the future.

Thirty Years of Progress on Food Safety

Over the past 30 years, Mayne said, data have enabled progress in shifting food safety from reactive to preventive efforts. She went on to describe microbial food safety, allergens in food, and chemical food safety as aspects of the food safety system.

Mayne explained that progress on microbial food safety includes the use of whole genome sequencing to detect and solve foodborne outbreaks and to identify root causes of pathogen contamination. For example, she said, this technology is used in food manufacturing facilities to determine whether a pathogen is resident or sporadic, a distinction that informs mitigation strategies. Sequenced pathogens have been sourced from food,

food facilities, and agricultural environments. Mayne noted that the GenomeTrakr Network hosts global data on pathogen sequences, and available data continue to grow exponentially (FDA, 2023). Established in 2013, she said, the GenomeTrakr Network had an average of 184 sequences added per month in the first year; in 2022, the average number of sequences added per month was 21,767. The database now holds more than 1.25 million pathogen sequences, with most the robust data for *Salmonella*, followed by *Escherichia coli (E. coli)/Shigella* and *Listeria monocytogenes*, Mayne reported.

Regarding progress on allergens in food, Mayne said that the Food Allergen and Labeling Consumer Protection Act of 2004 created the mandate that all food packages must contain labels listing priority allergens.[1] She stated that prior to that legislation, food manufacturers were not required to specify allergens on labels, so this constituted an important development for the food allergy community. Effective January 2023, the Food Allergen Safety, Treatment, Education, and Research Act of 2021 updated the list of priority allergens to include sesame.[2]

Outlining progress in food chemical safety, Mayne noted regulatory and industry efforts to reduce human exposure to chemicals of concern, including toxic elements, process-induced contaminants, and environmental contaminants. Regarding toxic elements, she noted that average daily lead intake in children aged 1–3 years has seen a dramatic decrease of 97 percent since 1980. Interventions to decrease lead exposure include removing lead from soldered cans, banning leaded gasoline, and implementing public health efforts, she said, and interventions to reduce exposure to process-induced contaminants include steps taken by the industry and FDA to reduce acrylamide, a chemical that can form in some foods when cooked at high temperatures. These efforts have resulted in a decline in mean acrylamide intake (FDA, n.d.), Mayne reported. Additionally, she continued, regulatory action targeting environmental contaminants such as dioxins, polychlorinated biphenyls, and certain per- and polyfluoroalkyl substances (PFAS) have led to substantial declines in exposure over recent decades. For example, National Health and Nutrition Examination Survey (NHANES) data indicate that blood levels of perfluorooctane sulfonate, a common PFAS, has decreased by more than 85 percent from 1999 to 2018 (ATSDR, 2024), Mayne said. She noted that other achievements in food safety include the development of hazard analysis critical control points

---

[1] Food Allergen and Labeling Consumer Protection Act of 2004, Public Law 108-282, Title II, 108th Cong., 2nd sess. (August 2, 2004).

[2] Food Allergy Safety, Treatment, Education, and Research Act of 2021, Public Law 117-11, 117th Cong., 1st sess. (April 23, 2021).

(HACCPs) and the focus on prevention generated by the FDA Food Safety Modernization Act (FSMA).[3]

Food Safety Considerations for the Future

Whole genome sequencing has the potential to expand more broadly, Mayne said, and FDA is working to develop the capacity to sequence viruses, such as hepatitis A and norovirus, and parasites, such as *Cyclospora cayetanensis*, that cause foodborne illness. She stated that global expansion of the GenomeTrakr Network—which currently contains data from laboratories in more than a dozen countries—is a priority, given the global nature of the U.S. food supply.

Mayne said that opportunities for progress in addressing allergens include determining allergen thresholds in foods with associated labeling to help food-allergic consumers; identifying new priority allergens and the criteria used to require priority allergen labeling; and facilitating international harmonization of priority allergens to address variance across countries.

In continuing to address the safety of chemicals in foods, Mayne stated that transparency is needed around domestic risk considerations, such as how FDA uses toxicity reviews and exposure evaluations to determine risk, especially given state legislation to ban particular food ingredients independent of FDA. Furthermore, Mayne noted, international variance in chemical risk determinations occurs when regulators in countries arrive at different conclusions on food chemical safety; this can engender confusion and lack of trust among consumers. Global harmonization on chemical risk determinations could help ameliorate consumer concerns. She added that a broader approach to consider chemical classes could avoid chemical "whack-a-mole," a practice in which industry responds to a chemical safety concern by moving to a different chemical that may have less toxicity data available than the chemical being phased out. Expanding the safety concern approach by including similar chemicals within a class could deter manufacturers from this practice, she said.

Mayne emphasized that more research—and research funding—is needed on pathogen prevalence and mitigation strategies in several key areas, including fresh produce. As examples, she mentioned that in recent years, *Cronobacter sakazakii* was found in powdered infant formula and data on prevalence are limited; and *E. coli* was found in flour—although flour is not a ready-to-eat food, outbreaks associated with flour occur.

While the ability to trace products within the food system is currently improving, Mayne said, more work remains to improve food traceability,

---

[3] FDA Food Safety Modernization Act, Public Law 111-353, 111th Cong., 2nd sess. (January 4, 2011).

supply chains, and recall effectiveness. An upcoming compliance date for the traceability rule has galvanized efforts in this area, yet not all foods are on the food traceability list. Broadly speaking, regulatory prioritization is needed to maximize impact, she suggested. Given the limited resources of regulatory agencies, Mayne continued, regulation should be driven by data mined effectively from a variety of sources, including artificial intelligence and machine learning. Global regulatory partnerships can increase efficient use of resources, and these partnerships can be based on comparability in food safety systems or based in comparability of food safety of selected commodities, such as the shrimp regulatory partnerships FDA is developing with certain countries. Mayne also called for additional surveillance and metrics efforts to ensure and assess progress in food safety. Because increased testing activities (of both cases and food) lead to greater detection of foodborne illness and more recalls, more aggressive food safety systems may reveal larger numbers of outbreaks and recalls. Thus, she explained, the quantity of outbreaks and recalls alone is not an accurate measure of food safety, so additional tools are needed.

Mayne underscored the need to anticipate and respond to challenges to food systems arising from climate change and global events such as the COVID-19 pandemic. During her recent 8-year tenure at FDA, extreme levels of flooding contaminated crops, which required FDA to determine whether these crops were safe to enter the human food supply. Pathogens such as *Vibrio vulnificus* that thrive in warm water are spreading to areas where they were not previously detected.

In addition to environmental challenges, Mayne said, innovation is changing the food landscape in areas such as cell-cultured foods, controlled environment agriculture, and food delivery models. She noted that regulatory efforts should support these innovations in food production and delivery while also ensuring safety. Moreover, she continued, consumer education needs to evolve in step with consumer food behaviors, address misinformation, and build knowledge and trust.

Mayne highlighted the relationship between nutrition and food safety with the example of *Listeria monocytogenes*, a pathogen for which 77 percent of food contamination in 2021 came from dairy products, vegetable row crops, and fruits. Given that U.S. dietary guidelines recommend these foods, safety measures are needed to support nutrition, she said. Mayne concluded by remarking that food safety progress (1) is enabled by partnerships between regulators, industry, academia, and consumers; (2) is fostered by data-driven technology that evolves over time; and (3) requires global partnerships for a safe global food supply.

MANUFACTURING PERSPECTIVE

Stefanie N. Evans, Conagra Brands, Inc., outlined advancements, challenges, and future directions of food safety from a manufacturing perspective. She noted that her career in food manufacturing began shortly after the *E. coli* outbreak within the Jack in the Box fast food chain in 1993, a landmark event that influenced her career choice. In the ensuing decades, she continued, substantial progress has been made through whole genome sequencing, bioinformatics, and source tracking.

Evans noted that the food industry uses modeling to examine how organisms behave in different types of environments, including food matrices, and continued advances in the modeling arena are possible. Furthermore, she said, data analytics have enabled decision making based on information and trends within food production facilities. Detection capabilities have progressed from basic traditional laboratory testing to innovative technology platforms based on DNA, she explained, thereby enabling much more rapid information, detection, and response to any contamination.

Evans remarked that knowledge of food safety issues has advanced over the past 30 years with the development of data on the prevalence of pathogens in various commodities, better understanding of how pathogens might travel through farming and facility environments, and the ability to map the movement of organisms. She highlighted the opportunity to further improve organism mapping. Advancement of mitigation techniques includes hurdle technologies that protect food and extend shelf life, Evans said, explaining that steps taken during processing increase food safety before packaging, and efforts in packaging environments inhibit the growth of potential hazards that could harm consumers. Technology in the food processing space has improved with more frequent use of high-pressure processing, which she said was formerly cost prohibitive for most manufacturers. Evans added that sous vide technology increases food safety. And, she said, alternative proteins have seen explosive growth over the past 10 years, with processing innovations driven by increased consumer interest in plant-based foods.

Current Food Safety Gaps and Challenges

A lack of investment in manufacturing and aging infrastructure—both in the United States and globally—slows the pace of applying food safety technology, Evans said. As an example, she said that scanning technology ensures that products match their packages and are thereby properly labeled; however, needed improvements in facility structures often supersede investment in scanning equipment.

Evans added that the adoption of food safety technology lags even in large companies. The food production workforce has become far more culturally diverse and experiences high turnover rates and labor shortages, she explained; these shifts pose challenges in adequately training employees who may be unfamiliar with safe manufacturing processes and who speak a variety of languages. For example, she said, one Conagra Brands facility employs workers speaking 15 different languages and multiple dialects. Efforts to meet training challenges include the use of electronic tablets, videos, and photos, and pairing less-experienced employees with more seasoned workers.

Safe agricultural practices and produce safety are additional areas in need of improvement, Evans remarked. Complicated supply chains in the context of globalization and e-commerce pose challenges to traceability, she said, given that many smaller companies within supply chains underfund digital and information technology (IT). Evans added that a lack of research in specific emerging organisms and in new technologies slows progress in food safety. Moreover, a gap in consumer education has enabled a consumer base disconnected from food origins and processes.

Potential for Advances in Food Safety

Evans highlighted numerous food technologies undergoing rapid development: a variety of alternative proteins; 3D printing; vertical, urban, and greenhouse farming; and genetically modified organisms (GMOs). Although developing technologies offer potential benefits, they also raise the possibility of food safety risks and hazards in a new context. For example, she said, contamination can occur even within the closed system of greenhouse farming. Furthermore, consumer education is crucial to communicate accurate information about the science of new technologies, and Evans underscored that poor consumer education efforts have contributed to misunderstandings about GMOs. Smart factories are creating new possibilities within the food manufacturing industry by collecting and integrating real-time digital information via electronic tablets on plant floors, she reported. But she said the adoption of such technology applications is slowed by the need to address aging infrastructure, which often needs to be prioritized over modernization efforts. Continued innovation is imperative, Evans stated, in order to address issues including globalization, resource depletion, sustainability, packaging, recycling, water reuse, climate change, carbon offsetting, and healthier diets. She noted that approaches to reusing water and recycling packaging can pose a risk of concentrating the very contaminants the industry seeks to reduce or eliminate.

Evans emphasized that a focus on fundamentals is critical for the food manufacturing industry; nine out of ten of the regulatory violations included in FDA Current Good Food Manufacturing Practices pertain to basic manufacturing practices that increase worker and product safety.

Investment in infrastructure is needed to create sanitary food production environments, she said. Continued labor challenges are expected, Evans continued, requiring automation and technology to ensure delivery of safe food; the food industry can capitalize on the ongoing development of digital tools to improve mapping and source tracking capabilities, which drive food safety. Additionally, she stated, the industry should continue to focus and improve upon detection, mitigation, and processing. Evans noted that the exciting opportunities offered by rapidly developing technology should not overshadow an emphasis on the day-to-day fundamentals of food safety delivery and consumer education efforts. She concluded by quoting a motto from the Food and Agriculture Organization of the United Nations: "Food safety is everyone's business." Evans defined *food safety* as a collective aim that encompasses simple actions such as handwashing, complex scientific evaluation of chemical compounds and pathogen isolation, robust governance, and data and information sharing.

FOOD SAFETY IN DEVELOPING ECONOMIES

Haley F. Oliver, U.S. Agency for International Development (USAID) Feed the Future Innovation Lab for Food Safety at Purdue University, outlined the implications of foodborne illnesses and opportunities to increase food safety in developing economies. She underscored that despite the advent of a global food supply, many people in the world continue to eat locally sourced food, and food safety is a ubiquitous need. Despite tremendous efforts from the regulatory and product sectors, foodborne disease persists, affecting one out of six Americans annually, Oliver reported, adding that notable foodborne diseases include norovirus, salmonellosis, campylobacteriosis, and toxoplasmosis. Globally, foodborne disease accounts for 600 million cases of illness and 420,000 deaths each year, while estimates of the cost associated with tracked foodborne pathogens exceed $15 billion, Oliver noted. The USAID investment in the Feed the Future Innovation Lab for Food Safety facilitates work linking food safety with food security. Oliver explained that when food is not safe, it no longer affords the benefits of food, and thus safety is a key component of food security in addition to nutrition, supply, and access. Foodborne illnesses drive malnutrition, carry potentially lifelong negative health implications, and create an economic burden, she said; however, foodborne illnesses are preventable, and prevention efforts aimed at establishing food safety in developing economies can remove barriers to economic growth and achieve global impact.

Oliver then described how foodborne pathogens interface with nutrition to create a cycle of disease and malnutrition. Unsafe food can lead to foodborne disease, she said, causing diarrhea and vomiting, and malabsorption of nutrients gives rise to malnutrition, stunting, and increased comorbidity. The dissemination of biological hazards into the environment compromises food safety, thus perpetuating the cycle, Oliver explained; therefore, disrupting this cycle improves nutrition.

Advancements in food safety in developing economies include aflatoxin prevention and awareness, as well as elevating understanding about chemical hazards, pesticides, and fertilizers as challenges to food safety, Oliver stated. She described a 2018 study conducted by the Global Food Safety Partnership that documents substantial investment in food safety programming in Africa focused on aflatoxins, pesticides, and fertilizers, she noted. However, she continued, the burden of foodborne disease remains linked to foodborne pathogens, indicating that better alignment between investment and health hazards may be beneficial. Oliver posited that the lack of investment in pathogen prevention in developing economies could be related to the difficulty in detecting bacteria, whereas mold on crops and the application of fertilizers and pesticides are readily observable.

Achieving Food Safety Goals in Developing Economies

Oliver summarized current challenges to achieving food safety goals within developing economies. Competing priorities—ranging from political concerns to climate issues to disease threats—impede the prioritization of food safety. Additionally, there are resource constraints within the United States as well as in global and developing economies. Confusion between safety and quality contributes to a lack of understanding that quality food can be unsafe, which in turn influences the effectiveness of policy. Gaps in infrastructure persist, particularly in the areas of inspection, cold chain, and testing laboratories. Education and personnel challenges create substantial barriers to food safety success. Regulatory structures differ between countries, as do the ramifications of foodborne illness, and these can affect the ability to meet food safety goals in developing economies.

Oliver explained how the Innovation Lab works to address these barriers through awareness, research, policy, and training. Awareness efforts focus on issues and effects of food safety and on measures to reduce food safety risks. Research investment targets include increasing local research capacity and conducting research on regional food safety challenges. New policy development and implementation of existing policies enable conditions for food safety research, translation, and practice. Training and education activities are designed to accelerate translational research technologies and practices.

Additional Considerations

Oliver noted a range of additional factors currently affecting food safety. The COVID-19 pandemic catalyzed increases in pathogen awareness, attention to food safety, consideration of labor hours, and investment in sanitation, she said. During the pandemic, *Listeria* prevalence in grocery stores decreased; however, Oliver reported, food safety behavior and practices have largely returned to the prepandemic status quo. Thus, human behavior and motivation are relevant research areas in determining how to increase food safety practices effectively, she said, adding that the pandemic also yielded insights into how food interfaces within hospital and long-term care systems. She suggested that diversity, equity, and inclusion aspects of food safety and security should be considered, to increase access to safe food. Cellular agriculture holds potential for addressing food security, but Oliver said that safety considerations of these foods should be analyzed before delivery into developing economies. She continued that the limitations of and improvements to disinfectants and sanitizers carry implications for the food industry, but prominent perspectives on disinfectants within developing economies may vary from those in the United States. For example, she said, acceptance of some of the most effective disinfectants, such as chlorine, is decreasing in some countries. She added that disease associated with low-moisture foods, such as infant formula and flour, requires greater research investment, particularly given the critical role of these food sources in food security.

DISCUSSION

The discussion following these presentations focused on infrastructure investment, multiple chemical exposures from food, regulation and innovation in food manufacturing, food safety and nutrition education in schools, maintaining food safety within a global supply chain, steps to address food allergens, and food traceability systems.

Investment in Infrastructure

Nugen noted the role of infrastructure in adoption of new technologies and asked about approaches to increasing investment in infrastructure within a context of low profit margins and consumer resistance to increased prices. Evans remarked that risk assessment is important in prioritizing investment in infrastructure according to associated risk. Mayne emphasized that old facilities and food manufacturing equipment pose significant challenges to sanitation and can create ongoing contamination issues, which in turn necessitate product disposal and recalls. Thus, she noted, manufacturers should consider such routine losses in revenue when determining whether to invest in upgraded facilities and equipment. Oliver stated that the percentage of the population consuming locally sourced food in developing economies can be as high as 90 percent; therefore, the technology needs in these settings differ from those in countries eating imported foods. For this reason, she said, the Innovation Lab is not investing in technology development, but focusing instead on creating environments that enable adoption of existing technologies and fostering the willingness to do so.

Multiple Chemical Exposures from Food

Kate Clancy, food systems consultant, asked about existing research or regulation on multiple exposures to chemicals or toxic agents from food. Mayne explained that chemicals within the same class in terms of structure can vary in how they affect pathways, with some stimulating a biochemical pathway and others slowing down that pathway, and with many chemicals affecting multiple chemical pathways. This level of complexity in science and data presents challenges to assessing whether multiple chemical exposures have similar versus opposing effects, she said. To address this, Mayne continued, FDA is using data mining and available technology to modernize toxicity evaluation, which will include an expanded decision tree currently under development. Evans remarked that in addition to a lack of data on multiple exposures, misinformation about chemicals and associated health hazards is often promoted on social media. This misinformation can detract from efforts to manage substances such as heavy metals and PFAS that pose known health hazards, she said. Evans added that state-by-state regulations, such as California's ban on some chemicals that are allowed in other states, complicate food manufacturing. Federal research and guidance could streamline approaches to chemical hazards. Oliver noted an opportunity for academia to address chemicals within food science and nutrition undergraduate programs.

Regulation and Innovation in Manufacturing

Barbara Schneeman, University of California, Davis, asked about the extent to which regulation facilitates and inhibits innovation in manufacturing; she asked specifically about regulations regarding infant formula notifications.[4] Mayne emphasized the importance of dialogue between regulators and the manufacturers considering innovation. For example,

---

[4] In 2022–2023, several U.S. companies initiated voluntary recalls of infant formula after detecting *Cronobacter sakazakii* in their products, leading to nationwide supply shortages.

she said, communication between industry and subject matter experts at FDA began early in the process of developing cell-cultured foods and included facility tours to demonstrate how these foods would be made. This type of discussion supports innovation while ensuring it can be achieved safely, Mayne stated. Regarding infant formula notifications, she continued, companies considering changes in manufacturing processes should consult with FDA—a significant change in the manufacturing of infant formula could affect a sole source of nutrition for many infants, and the regulatory perspective could benefit infant formula companies. Evans remarked on industry collaboration with FDA and the U.S. Department of Agriculture (USDA), particularly regarding FSMA regulations, noting that this collaboration declined during the COVID-19 pandemic. In developing systems for the adoption of new technologies, such as high-pressure processing, Evans said, Conagra Brands communicates with and provides data to FDA. She stated that rather than being an impediment to innovation, collaboration between industry and regulators establishes shared knowledge and facilitates the approval process. Oliver commented that manufacturers encounter additional costs in meeting increased regulatory requirements, and that greater investment in food—which is relatively inexpensive in the United States—may be necessary to improve safety within food systems.

Food Safety and Nutrition Education

Isabel Walls, USDA, asked about the promotion of food safety and nutrition education in schools. Mayne noted that FDA developed curricula about food safety, entitled "Science and Our Food Supply," that middle and high school science teachers can adopt. She remarked that scientific literacy, a growing challenge in the United States, contributes to the spread of misinformation and lack of consumer trust. Given the abundance of conflicting information, she continued, many consumers determine that no information is trustworthy; therefore, decreasing science literacy undermines scientific efforts to improve food safety and public health. Evans emphasized the need for more safety education in schools and beyond, citing the Partnership for Food Safety Education's efforts to educate adults via social media. She stated that the Food Forum could focus on the need for food safety education, particularly within the context of changing food procurement avenues, including farmers' markets, community-supported agriculture, and e-commerce vendors that ship perishable food ingredients directly to consumers—a method that is vulnerable to temperature abuse. Mayne added that the Conference for Food Protection and FDA collaborated to create guidelines for food sold through e-commerce, but greater dissemination and awareness of these guidelines is needed. Oliver commented that the National Association of State Departments of Agriculture is a potential mechanism for advocating for educational components to be added into state curricula. Teaching food safety behaviors to younger generations could result in change that lasts throughout their lifetime, she said.

Food Safety Within a Global Food Supply Chain

Ajay P. Malshe, Purdue University, asked about the role of supply chains in the food safety system, given that the supply chain has become global and that bacterial growth may occur in the interfaces in manufacturing and supply chain. Mayne described how FSMA has established standards that apply to food and ingredients imported from other countries, as well as to food that is entirely domestically manufactured. However, the tools and levers for achieving food safety vary, she said; for example, FSMA established the Foreign Supplier Verification Program (FSVP), which places the onus on importers to ensure that food safety mandates are met by suppliers. She highlighted a recent incident in which U.S. children became sick with lead poisoning after eating applesauce containing cinnamon imported from Ecuador. Under FSMA, the safety of all ingredients and the final product should have been ensured, preventing such incidents, but this mandate was not met, she said. A lack of preventive controls and good manufacturing practices can lead to unsafe ingredients, which Evans said underscores the importance of adhering to standards throughout the supply chain. She stated that education efforts are needed to help small and medium-sized companies understand what FSVP entails and how to build programs to ensure compliance. Evans said that outside of the large consumer packaging goods companies that were heavily involved with FSMA regulations, a thorough understanding of FSVP is lacking. She added that regulatory FSVP inspections are likely lacking at smaller companies. Conagra Brands created an international team that audits and inspects facilities in an effort to drive food safety while protecting global supply chains, Evans reported. Given the variance in worldwide food safety standards, she said, ensuring safety of imported ingredients is a complex process. Moreover, Evans pointed out, recent inflation in the cost of goods could contribute to a potential increase in food adulteration.

Addressing Food Allergens

Robert Earl, Food Allergy Research and Education, asked about the advancement of education, protections, and labeling for people with food allergies. By reducing the intentional addition of food allergens and facilitating the adoption of food allergen thresholds, Earl continued, the safe food supply for the food allergy population would increase. Mayne emphasized that the leading cause of food recall in the United States is undeclared allergens, and mislabeled product constitutes an extensive problem requiring solutions. Consumers with food allergies have asked for allergen thresholds, Mayne said, because statements that a product may contain an allergen or was manufactured in a facility that also uses an allergen are vague for the purposes of informed decision making. Efforts to establish allergen thresholds are currently underway via the Codex Alimentarius international food standards, she explained. Should research reveal a de minimis level of an allergen that can be tolerated, along with appropriate food labeling, additional foods could become available to consumers with food allergies, Mayne stated. Evans remarked on the need for changes regarding allergens, as some companies opt to label products as potentially containing allergens rather than establishing procedures to control allergens. She explained that efficient removal of allergenic proteins from facilities is feasible; in fact, most manufacturing issues with allergens arise from products being incorrectly placed in packaging intended for other products. Technology could decrease mislabeling by ensuring that products and packaging are accurately matched, Mayne said; scanning technology is advancing quickly, having evolved from bar codes to two-dimensional matrices. However, she said, adoption of technology advancements is often impeded by the need to prioritize infrastructure investment. Oliver noted that she collaborates with people in developing economies who communicate that allergens are not a problem in their countries. A lack of awareness around allergens could translate into ingredient production and affect the global supply chain, she continued. Evans commented that equipment is often used for multiple types of agricultural commodities—for example, a truck may be used to transport both soy and wheat—posing allergen risks to supply chains. Thus, she said, establishing allergen thresholds would bolster supply chain risk assessment.

Food Traceability Systems

Naomi K. Fukagawa, USDA Beltsville Human Nutrition Research Center, asked about the status of blockchain food traceability. Evans replied that a lack of robust investment in data platforms throughout a supply chain poses challenges to adoption of blockchain food traceability systems. Even large companies that invest in IT platforms, such as Conagra Brands, face tracing challenges, she said; these challenges tend to increase for small suppliers, particularly those in low-income countries where records are often kept manually and on paper. Mayne noted that traceability is limited to the data available, highlighting a need for investment in data platforms; and she said that multiple technologies, including blockchain, can enable traceability. Food manufacturers often cite the cost of traceability as pro-hibitively high, which led FDA to sponsor a low- or no-cost traceability challenge that invited developers to submit ideas for low-cost traceability systems, Mayne said. In approximately 2 years, she continued, FDA will require compliance in tracing certain foods on a food traceability list; it mandates traceability for foods that pose the highest food safety risks. However, she said, as companies establish systems to trace these foods, they are likely to extend these systems to the other foods they produce. Mayne cautioned that it will require substantial efforts to achieve the traceability needed to accurately track outbreaks to root causes throughout highly complex supply chains. Oliver added that a food system workforce with the requisite data science skills will be required to generate the data needed for traceability—a capacity that is currently limited.

4

Food Systems and Sustainability

The third session of the symposium featured three presentations and a discussion on the role of research, industry, and approaches to change in creating sustainable food systems that address pressing issues such as climate change, obesity, and diet-related chronic diseases. The session was moderated by Christina Khoo, Ocean Spray Cranberries, Inc.

FOOD SYSTEMS RESEARCH AND CLIMATE CHANGE

Jessica Fanzo, Food for Humanity Initiative at Columbia University, discussed the emerging climate change crisis and suggested strategies that can be undertaken by food systems researchers to address it. Sustainability in food systems encapsulates environmental, social, and economic sustainability, and notable advancements have been made within food systems over the past 30 years (Wood et al., 2023). For instance, there is now greater alignment regarding what constitutes a healthy diet, she said, and efforts led by the Food and Agriculture Organization and the U.S. government have improved accuracy in estimating the number of people experiencing hunger, elucidated the underlying issues fueling hunger, and revealed inequities. Recent decades have seen considerable food systems research and the amplification of that research into action. Fanzo remarked on the accelerating influence of thorough science on public health policy, exemplified by research-informed worldwide efforts to reduce trans fats. Moreover, she stated, the food system can now be advanced to new frontiers—such as the microbiome, the proliferation of ultra-processed foods and associated detriment to human health, and alternative proteins.

It is now widely acknowledged that food systems sit at the center of human and planetary health; in this context, Fanzo emphasized the critical need to address climate change. Describing the uncertainty about the future that persists despite the wealth of knowledge humans have amassed, she quoted Joan Didion (1968), who wrote, "It's easy to see the beginnings of things, and harder to see the ends." Lessons from history should inform action, she maintained; for example, the National Aeronautics and Space Administration failed to heed warnings ahead of the launch of the space shuttle *Challenger*, which resulted in catastrophe. For more than 40 years, Fanzo said, scientists have informed the U.S. government about human contributions to climate change, yet little action has been taken. She suggested that the current spate of extreme weather events related to climate change supports the statement that "the risks of making well-intentioned but inappropriate policy choices are much smaller than the risks of using a lack of evidence as an argument for inaction" (Rich, 2018).

Fanzo highlighted the active role that food systems researchers should play in addressing the climate change crisis. She summarized perspectives on needed changes to food systems and steps the food systems research community should take in creating sustainability, citing the numerous arguments and narratives at play regarding the direction needed for food systems (Béné et al., 2019): Agronomists would tend to prioritize greater calorie production through increases in crops and yields, but the nutrition community might contend that the nutrient gap must be closed by diversifying food supply and production systems. The social justice community focuses on the need for greater equity, sovereignty, and food autonomy across food systems by shifting the global food system to more localized systems, and environmentalists prioritize protecting landscapes and consideration of ecosystem services and natural resources in food production. Such variance in narratives, priorities, and values culminates in a highly fractured governing mechanism for food systems, said Fanzo. She urged that researchers continue to fill gaps in knowledge to increase understanding of how food systems affect diets, nutrition, and health outcomes in various contexts, with different drivers, and in relation to political and societal transitions (Fanzo et al., 2021). Moreover, Fanzo stated, it is important for researchers to bolster an understanding of the potential implications of the current and future food systems for the environment and overall planetary health. She asserted that the generation of evidence should consider the role of nutrition in environmental sustainability to better understand the bidirectional relationship between the environment and human diet, nutrition, and health. And, she said, research efforts should extend beyond understanding effects to identifying levers of change within food systems—which may pertain to politics, data, communication, or other drivers—and learning how to effectively operate these levers.

Fanzo and colleagues (2021) developed a roadmap for research at the intersection of food systems, the environment, and nutrition to address various research methods, intervention points, and goals of intervention. Nutrition research methods include basic science research, clinical research, epidemiology, implementation science, inquiry into lived experiences, systems science, transdisciplinary research, and meta research. Fanzo stated that these research methods intersect with points of intervention throughout the food system involving nutrients, human biology, dietary patterns, human behavior, food environments, food supply chains, and production practices. Achieving the goals of these interventions will entail challenging, transdisciplinary work that requires collaboration and collective problem-solving efforts, she asserted. Adding to the challenge, societal shifts have created a dynamic in which scientific facts and evidence are under great scrutiny and sometimes openly disregarded as suspect by politicians and business leaders. Noting that research has played a vital role in charting a positive and sustainable direction for global food security, nutrition, and health, she emphasized that the rigors of science and evidence must be maintained. Research holds the potential to bring about wholesale changes in attitudes, political thought, and action, she said.

Fanzo outlined factors involved in social change and noted inherent challenges. She offered the example of the United Nations Climate Change Conference of Parties (COP), which took 27 years to bring fossil fuels into negotiations and to date has yet to address food systems. Change involves policy, she said, so it is important for researchers to consider approaches to motivate policymakers to engage in systems thinking. In addition to generating evidence, researchers should share data and encourage policymakers to use it, Fanzo urged; to this end, researchers should ensure that evidence is useful. To galvanize political will and action, she suggested that researchers empower people who work in food systems and amplify their voices. Additionally, she said, the food space should be negotiated in climate agendas and incentives should be put in place to motivate actors, the private sector, and governments to act on food systems. She emphasized that time is of the essence, as only a decade remains in which to stop the increased warmth of the planet before the initiation of natural processes that will raise temperatures further. Fanzo emphasized that this calls for bold action to foster global citizenry and sustainability. Although daunting, these challenges can be met, she said, offering the example of the plains bison, which were slaughtered nearly to the point of extinction. Once numbering in the tens of millions, the plains bison population decreased to less than 1,000 by the late 1880s. Yet, she recalled, conservation efforts have succeeded in increasing the population to more than 350,000, highlighting the ability of humans to course-correct when they summon the will and courage to act.

THE HEALTH AND SUSTAINABILITY JOURNEY
OF DANONE NORTH AMERICA

Stephanie K. Goodwin, Danone North America, discussed Danone's industry approach to generating solutions for creating a healthy, resilient, and sustainable food system. Danone is a global food manufacturer that started as a European yogurt company more than a century ago. In the 1940s, Danone began selling yogurt in small, single-serving porcelain jars in New York pharmacies. In the decades since, Goodwin said, Danone has grown into a global business that sells dairy yogurt, plant-based food and beverages, coffee, water, and medical foods through brands such as Dannon, Oikos, Dugro, Activia, Horizon, Silk, and So Delicious. The company works toward the mission of bringing health through food to as many people as possible. Danone's vision is "one planet, one health," based on the belief that the health of the planet and the health of people are inextricably linked. Therefore, ensuring that healthy food is accessible by all requires a healthy planet with strong ecosystems that exist in harmony with resilient social structures.

Goodwin described how Danone has created business models that leverage their corporate activity in realizing its vision. One of the largest certified B corporations in the world, Danone has a legal obligation to protect and consider effects on all key players, rather than on shareholders alone, she stated, which entails promoting a model of sustainable growth that creates economic and social value for customers, employees, and suppliers while improving environmental impact. Infusing this purpose through governance structure, brand, strategy, metrics, and future planning, Danone developed a roadmap for sustainable, profitable growth and value creation, Goodwin explained. The roadmap is a concrete, measurable framework that clarifies health and sustainability priorities within the pillars of health, nature, and people and communities, she said, priorities that are translated into mid- to long-term objectives and key performance indicators (KPIs) to maintain focus on creating positive effects on the health of people and the planet.

Goodwin outlined roadmap objectives for the next 7 years within the health pillar. She said that at the 2022 White House Conference on Hunger, Nutrition, and Health, Danone North America (NA) committed to investing $22 million toward building healthy, sustainable dietary patterns that will contribute to reducing hunger, food insecurity, and diet-related diseases. This commitment involves action toward White House–specified goals that include improving food access and affordability, empowering all consumers to make and have access to healthy food choices, enhancing nutrition and food security research, and integrating nutrition and health, Goodwin said. To improve food access and affordability, she noted, Danone

NA agreed to support federal feeding programs (e.g., the Special Supplemental Nutrition Program for Women, Infants, and Children), collaborate with community organizations (e.g., Green Bronx Machine and City Harvest), and commission a study on the state of nutrition quality in the United States. This study indicated that nutrition has become a top priority on the U.S. agenda, Goodwin stated, with access to quality food ranked as one of the most important current issues alongside the economy, jobs, and health care. Integrating nutrition and health involves a company focus on improving the nutrition profile of Danone products, she said. To empower consumers in accessing and choosing healthy foods, Danone NA partners with organizations and retailers to conduct several education campaigns targeting consumers and health care providers. Goodwin highlighted that the company enhances nutrition and food security research by providing funds and grants for studying health and nutrition research topics. She said that Danone NA's efforts to integrate nutrition and health focus on enhancing the product portfolio by driving nutrition density and reducing added sugar, with a specific focus on the nutrition of children's products and plant-based products with low or no added sugar. To date, Goodwin reported, the company has launched new low- or no-added-sugar products and has various innovations and reformulations currently underway. Given that consumers choose products that they enjoy eating, she said, Danone is working to improve nutrient density while ensuring that products have appealing flavor and texture.

Goodwin described Danone's roadmap efforts within the nature pillar, which include a focus on regenerative agriculture. As a set of farming practices that protect soil, water, and biodiversity, regenerative agriculture respects animal welfare, acknowledges the role of farmers and positive effects of farming, and considers factors related to economic viability. Core regenerative agriculture practices help to restore ecosystems, mitigate climate change, and ensure resilient agrifood systems. In support of climate-smart agriculture, Goodwin said, Danone NA has partnered with the U.S. Department of Agriculture (USDA) to provide $70 million in climate-smart commodities grants focused primarily on dairy, oats, and soy. Goodwin outlined grant objectives that include reducing dairy methane gas emissions, creating infrastructure to sustainably grow and trace U.S. oats, and building capacity for processing both traceable food-grade and organic soy for dairy feed.

Goodwin summarized considerations for the future of food systems. Public–private partnerships should be established and scaled to meet current challenges, she stated. Companies should be familiar with all components of their supply chains and work directly with farmers to improve the long-term economic resilience of farms. Goodwin said that improvements can be accomplished through partnerships with third parties, with new technology, and by using in-depth field-level analysis and goal setting. However, she pointed out, these improvements entail cost, time, and technology burdens for farmers, third parties, and the industry, all of which will need to be addressed. Appropriate education and information should be made accessible to all parties, and industry alignment is needed on standards and methodologies used, she added.

Given that an improved system is only useful if adopted, Danone NA is involved in collaborative efforts to develop sustainable nutrition, said Goodwin. Danone NA participates in and sponsors the Tufts University Food and Nutrition Innovation Council, which convenes a Sustainable Nutrition working group. Bringing together representatives from industry, academia, and nonprofit organizations, Goodwin explained, the working group seeks to find common goals and workstreams at the intersection of nutrition and environmental sustainability. It envisions a global food system that provides equitable access to sufficient, safe, nutritious, affordable, and culturally relevant food for everyone; moreover, Goodwin continued, this food system prioritizes taste and palatability while simultaneously improving the long-term sustainability and resilience of the planet and health of the global population. Ultimately, the group intends to inform policy by developing science-based recommendations, guidelines, and strategies, she explained.

Goodwin acknowledged that the process of determining priorities and initial focal points among industry, academics, and nonprofit organizations is complex. Furthermore, she stated, both top-down and bottom-up support for sustainable nutrition food systems are needed to generate adequate change. Goodwin asserted that consumers primarily choose food based on taste and price, and environmental impact does not necessarily factor into consumer selection. Rather than waiting on customers to demand sustainable foods, the food industry must offer customers a vision of healthy, regenerative, and resilient food systems, she maintained. This will warrant the creation of standards, frameworks, mapping exercises, evaluation, and communication of progress to business leadership, investors, government, and consumers, Goodwin said. Instead of responding to calls for change from government and nonprofit organizations, she urged, the food industry should lead the charge in proactively working toward positive change through the adoption of climate-smart policies and standards. Realizing the vision of sustainable food systems will require collaboration across sectors and throughout the supply chain, she said, and needed change entails recognizing that financial investment will create long-term benefits for the planet; human health; and businesses, including farms. The increasing prevalence of climate change effects, obesity, and diet-related chronic diseases strengthens the case for nutritious diets sourced from sustainable and resilient food systems. Goodwin asserted that actions taken within the next 5 years will affect human well-being for the next 30 years; thus, she said, the current moment is an opportunity to evolve, create more resilient business models, develop relevant brands, and join forces with all key players to accelerate sustainable and resilient food nutrition systems.

SUSTAINABILITY RESEARCH AND CHANGE PROCESSES

Christian Peters, USDA Agricultural Research Service, explored frameworks and approaches for understanding and addressing sustainability-related needs. He outlined a framework for assessing effects of the food system that centers on a supply chain connected to the spheres of science and technology, social organizations, biophysical environment, policies, and markets (Meadows, 2008). The concept of food systems encompasses the physical components of the food supply chain as well as the other independent systems involved. Entry of this interconnected food systems concept into the mainstream reflects increased application of systems thinking, Peters remarked. Moreover, he said, progress has been achieved in measuring environmental sustainability indicators, which enable sophisticated data analysis. Peters gave the example of researchers who have estimated emissions from the food system at the global scale, partitioned emissions into various gases, and attributed these to different sectors and stages of the food system (Crippa et al., 2021). The ability to put environmental sustainability indicators into context has also advanced, he said, as exemplified by the planetary boundaries concept, which uses a radar diagram to show various areas of impact, such as climate change, land use, freshwater use, biochemical flows, and ocean acidification (Steffen et al., 2015). The effects are coded green, yellow, or red according to whether the effect is within safe boundaries, is at an increasing risk of exceeding safe boundaries, or is at high risk of exceeding safe boundaries, respectively. This model can simultaneously apply to varied impact measures to consider total effects within specific areas, Peters added. Furthermore, he continued, the ability to extend this approach beyond the environment is advancing, thus enabling the concurrent modeling of multiple dimensions of sustainability.

Peters discussed food systems goals and associated effects on sustainability. From 1990 to 2015, global greenhouse gas emissions from food systems increased 42 percent, whereas emissions from developing countries increased by 101 percent and emissions from industrialized nations decreased by 6 percent (Crippa et al., 2021, Fig. 2). He noted that population growth in low-income countries likely contributes to increasing emissions. The lack of progress toward food system sustainability is due to current priorities and dynamics, Peters stated. The food supply chain comprises primary production, processing, food distribution, food service, and consumers. Along this supply chain, food and food services move upstream from production to consumers, and money and demand move downstream from consumers to production. Over the course of the twenty-first century, Peters explained, U.S. food systems have been driven by the goals of making food more abundant and more affordable. He said that efforts toward increased food production include yield-improving technologies, agricultural genetics, and management improvements. Labor-saving technology is used throughout the supply chain to increase the efficiency of food production, which in turn increases both food supply and affordability, he noted. Peters reported that more recent goals seek to produce an adequate, affordable food supply within ecological boundaries to promote sustainability, support balanced nutrition in the hopes of improving human health, and provide economic development through job creation. Consequently, more is being asked of the food system; Peters asserted that change is needed to achieve these broader goals.

Peters outlined leverage points for shifting the food system toward sustainability. *Thinking in Systems: A Primer* by Donella H. Meadows (2008) identifies 12 leverage points for shifting systems, three of which are particularly relevant to changes needed in food systems, Peters said. He explained that goals relate to the purpose or function of the system and constitute a leverage point when goals are changed to improve system outcomes. Paradigms form the mindset from which a system arises, he said, and changing paradigms—and by extension, changing mindsets—can change a system. Even more powerful, he noted, transcending paradigms is a leverage point that can be used by detaching from a fixed mindset about the food system. Peters acknowledged that while these three leverage points arguably have the greatest ability to affect change, they are also the most difficult leverage points to shift. Yet, he asserted, creating a sustainable, nutritious, adequate, and affordable food system that provides economic development opportunities will involve changing goals and mindsets, making needed change inherently challenging.

Peters provided a research perspective on steps to take in approaching such change. Applied research is appropriate in this endeavor because of its generality and applicability at multiple scales, he said. And, he continued, building consensus through applied research toward new food system goals and mindsets involves asking compelling questions with broad appeal and pursuing these questions collaboratively. Bringing key players together and asking questions that many people agree are important can be effective, Peters asserted, even in circumstances in which the group does not necessarily agree on the answers and may have strong preconceived notions about the answers. Included key players should represent various research disciplines as well as positions in the food system that are not focused on research full time. When consideration of complex problems leads to fragmented focus, returning to goals and first principles can reorient problem-solving to a shared vision, remarked Peters.

DISCUSSION

The discussion following the presentations focused on addressing food system problem areas in working toward sustainability, decreasing food system contributions to climate change, amplifying food safety and nutrition within sustainability efforts, the intersection of the health care and food systems, and approaches to overcoming reluctance of leaders to call for short-term sacrifices that yield long-term benefits.

Areas to Address in Achieving Sustainability

Khoo highlighted the need to support food systems' sustainability and farmers' livelihoods simultaneously. She asked about scaling successful efforts and collaboratively addressing problem areas in working toward sustainable food systems. Peters commented on the challenge of conducting interdisciplinary research when lacking both funds and the ability to convene researchers. Engaging a variety of key players requires time and resources that are currently lacking, he said. Fanzo remarked that technology has enabled progress toward global food security—for example, the Green Revolution successfully reduced famines through improvements in seeds, rows, and infrastructure. However, she said, the Green Revolution and the use of technology have bred unintended consequences. Fanzo emphasized that issues related to the use, access, justice, and unintended consequences of technology have led some people to believe that a more holistic systems approach is needed, one in which community social adhesion is matched with technology and improved policy. A biofortified crop is a tool in creating adequate food supply, but it will be insufficient in contending with massive burdens of malnutrition, inequities, and social injustices, Fanzo contended. Goodwin remarked that the complexity of the food system has historically received insufficient attention. She asserted that a system that involves food safety, nutrition, health, employees, land, and environmental impact should be approached with understanding of the interconnectedness throughout the system and about the system's effects on the planet and on the future.

Decreasing Food System Contributions to Climate Change

Josh Anthony, Nlumn, emphasized that a mere decade remains before conditions potentially reach a point at which climate change can no longer be reversed by human efforts. Given the complex and multidimensional nature of addressing sustainability, he asked, which sectors could achieve the most meaningful impact? Fanzo replied that the global food system uses substantial fossil fuel resources and contributes approximately 30 percent of total greenhouse gases, with the remaining 70 percent emitted by the energy, transportation, and building sectors. She reported that research from the University of Oxford outlines three major steps that, taken simultaneously, could prevent the food system from being a major contributor to reaching an increase of 1.5 degrees Celsius in global temperatures—in other words, the point at which climate change effects would potentially become irreversible: (1) decreasing food waste by half, as approximately 30 percent of all food produced is currently wasted; (2) making farm management more sustainable, including reducing the methane emitted by cows and rice, two major sources of methane; and (3) shifting toward plant-dominant diets for humans, particularly in locations where meat is consumed daily. Together, Fanzo said, these three efforts hold promise in dramatically decreasing the food system's contributions to climate change. Although a range of policy tools and industry incentives could be used to stimulate action in these areas, governments are reluctant to address diet, she noted. While politicians may speak of methane reduction or minimizing food loss, they rarely mention changes to diet because of associated issues of autonomy and self-liberty. Fanzo concluded that while multiple simultaneous actions are needed, governments are hesitant to take on such efforts.

Goodwin remarked that to address the scale of efforts needed, the food industry should partner with scientists and third parties to set clear, measurable standards, KPIs, and metrics that can be applied across the industry to measure impact. All parts of the supply chain must work toward sustainability, she maintained, and each company should work within its supply chain to comply with the specific standards developed for the industry. Peters acknowledged that moving toward sustainability will involve winners and losers, a dynamic that breeds contention and can pose barriers to progress.

Amplifying Nutrition and Food Safety

Caitlin Boon, Mars, Inc., described Mars as a company dedicated to sustainability, as evidenced by COP participation and release of a roadmap for achieving net-zero greenhouse gas emissions by 2050. She asked how nutrition and food safety can be amplified within the sustainability discussion, given the limited avenues and forums for such issues. Goodwin emphasized the value of inviting multidisciplinary expertise into discussions by ensuring that nutrition, food safety, food systems, and agriculture are represented. Additionally, she said, scenarios of food systems change can be modeled to determine potential ramifications, including macroeconomics and geopolitical effects, thereby enabling identification of scenarios on which multidisciplinary key players are willing to align. Peters noted that multidisciplinary discussion fosters broader consideration of factors by bringing together experts in various fields. Fanzo highlighted that the summer of 2023 was illuminating for many governments because it was the hottest summer on record and the coldest summer expected from a future perspective. The summer brought heat waves, wildfires, floods, and droughts throughout the world. Extreme climate-related events can generate water and food insecurity, food safety issues, and lack of shelter, she said. Governments fear scenarios in which they cannot feed, hydrate, and shelter their citizens, and, Fanzo asserted, such considerations of extreme events bring food safety and nutrition into the climate agenda. The effects of climate change are no longer hypothetical, she continued, and the worldwide experience of climate variability involves food safety, nutrition, and food security. Therefore, engagement with communities and governments contending with extreme events provides opportunities to address these issues.

Intersection of Health Care and Food Systems

Cheryl Toner, American Heart Association, emphasized that the health care sector is a key player in food systems, noting efforts by her organization and other entities to forge stronger connections between the food and health care systems. She asked about food system challenges and opportunities related to health care system engagement. Fanzo replied that many professionals in the food sector began their careers in the health sector: Nutrition connects these spaces. She noted that the field of international nutrition involves communication with ministers of health and of agriculture; however, nutrition is often neglected by both ministries. The COVID-19 pandemic was an extreme global health event that affected other systems including food, economics, and education, bringing attention to the interdependence of systems and highlighting the need to consider how those systems affect one another. Goodwin remarked that the intersection of nutrition and health care generally has long-term effects, such as reduction in chronic disease. The pandemic generated immediate effects of the health system on the food system, as well as acute awareness of these interactions, she said. This awareness launched the Food Is Medicine movement, she noted, providing an opportunity to bring together representatives from this movement, health care, agriculture, and environmental sustainability to participate in multidisciplinary problem-solving. Peters commented that the current food supply would not support universal alignment of individual diets with dietary guidelines. The food supply is, in part, a reflection of the foods that consumers buy. Thus, additional social aspects—such as the effect of poverty on food access—should be considered in identifying the barriers to creating a nutritious, affordable food supply, Peters remarked.

Approaching Short-Term Sacrifices for Long-Term Benefits

Guy Poppy, UK Research and Innovation, commented that issues related to climate change and food systems tend to be chronic but punctuated by occasional emergency or extreme events. Addressing chronic issues can involve changes that take time to yield benefit and cause short-term disadvantages, he said. For this reason, he pointed out, many politicians seeking reelection and business leaders trying to satisfy shareholders may be unwilling to make changes toward long-term benefit. He asked about approaches to needed change within the context of this dynamic. Goodwin remarked that the dynamic renders reliance on government policy for needed change inadequate; instead, industry can lead the charge by ushering in change. She said that businesses that make needed improvements can serve as models for other companies and as proof that sustainability and economic growth are not mutually exclusive. Fanzo emphasized that policymakers tend to think in terms of the cost of change and the financial return on investment, and extreme weather events carry a high financial cost; thus, an economic argument can be made in moving toward sustainability. The Infrastructure Investment and Jobs Act offers an example of U.S. willingness to invest in longer-term sustainability, she said.[1] Simultaneously, grassroots support for sustainability and accountability for climate change is increasing and is particularly evident in youth activism. Although U.S. activism has not focused on the food system, Fanzo continued, farmers in India and South America have held protests. Populations disproportionately affected by climate change—such as African Americans, Native Americans, women, and youth—have an opportunity to unify and apply pressure on the government to correct these inequities, she said. Fanzo emphasized that protests need to reach a much larger scale to influence government action. Peters noted that using familiar analogies and examples, such as saving for retirement, can help people understand the value of short-term sacrifice in achieving long-term benefit.

---

[1] Infrastructure Investment and Jobs Act, Public Law 117-58, 117th Cong., 1st sess. (November 15, 2021).

5

Nutrition and Health

The fourth session of the symposium featured three presentations and a discussion on the role of personalized nutrition, food composition, and equity considerations in nutrition and health. The session was moderated by Christina Khoo, Ocean Spray Cranberries, Inc.

THE PROMISE OF PERSONALIZED NUTRITION

Josh Anthony, Nlumn, discussed the role of personalized nutrition in creating an affordable, accessible, and acceptable food system that helps every individual make better choices and live a healthier life. Nlumn is a consulting company that assists businesses in participating more fully in the personalized nutrition and precision health marketplace. *Personalized nutrition* uses individual, specific information founded in evidence-based science to promote dietary behavior change that may result in measurable health benefits (Adams et al., 2020; Ordovas et al., 2018). Anthony described a cycle of four components—benefits, measurement, information, and behavior change—that create a workable, minimal, viable ecosystem. Specific benefits are related to the problem being addressed. Measurement involves tracking objective and credible metrics of health or function benefit, and Anthony explained that these measurements yield information that should empower users to improve their health and lifestyle, thereby affecting behavior change. In turn, he said, behavior change offers benefit, and the cycle continues.

Anthony outlined system-wide implications of health issues in the United States and technological advances that create a foundation for personalized health approaches. He reported that the nation spends more than $4 trillion on annual health care costs, 90 percent of which are for chronic illnesses and mental health (Buttorff et al., 2023). Poor health has dramatic effects on worker productivity, resulting in more than $550 billion in annual costs to U.S. employers (Japsen, 2020), Anthony said, noting that this figure surpasses the annual revenue of Microsoft, Amazon, or Apple. Poor health also increases mortality rates, he said, and preventive care could save approximately 100,000 U.S. lives each year. Anthony asserted that personalization can drive preventive care and that technological advancements are making more personalized approaches possible. Over the past 30 years, he related, several technology innovations have enabled the rise of personalized approaches. Sequencing of the human genome from 1990 to 2003 led to a bold vision for "P4 medicine" (i.e., medicine that is predictive, preventive, personalized, and participatory) (Japsen, 2020; NHGRI, 2023). In 1992, IBM announced the first smartphone, and in 2007 Apple revolutionized the industry with the launch of the iPhone, enabling people to carry personal computers in their pockets. Smartphones are an unmatched source of social and behavioral data, Anthony remarked, and the challenge of translating these data into behavior change persists. In 1994, the rise of metabolomics began with experiments that combined liquid chromatography and mass spectroscopy. The development and commercialization of microarrays have furthered the field, he said, and the metabolome, proteome, and lipidome can now be examined in combination with genomics. Computational biology yields insights into the systems of biology, standing in sharp contrast to the reductionist approach to biology that was common in decades prior. The Massachusetts Institute of Technology developed smart clothes, augmented reality, and wearable devices in the late 1990s, and Seiko launched the first "smart watch" during the same period. Currently, Anthony continued, approximately 60 million people track health statistics with a smart watch or similar device. In 2019, he said, artificial intelligence (AI) advanced with the development of generative, pretrained transformer models capable of generating coherent and contextually relevant sentences and could search and analyze disparate datasets. Anthony stated that this new level of AI capability shifts approaches to biological data algorithms and holds promise in integrating behavioral data to propel efforts to change health outcomes.

Anthony acknowledged that, despite technical advancements, the ability to demonstrate efficacy in personalized nutrition is in the early stages. In this context, he said, *efficacy* refers to the ability to deliver health and functional benefits that can be maintained over time and are better than population-based guidelines (NHGRI, 2023). Anthony remarked that demonstrating efficacy will involve overcoming numerous challenges—for instance, assessing the ability of personalized nutrition to deliver health and functional benefits requires (1) simple and reliable measures of nutrient status to establish baseline and progress; (2) a clear definition of the continuum of disease to health; and (3) identification of biomarker combinations that predict disease. Demonstrating that results are better than population-based guidelines, which are measured by the absence of disease, will require more representative datasets and experimental approaches, such as single-subject studies, he said. Showing that outcomes can be maintained over time involves longitudinal studies, which are often difficult and expensive, stated Anthony. Additionally, he explained, an individual's health needs change over time, and achievement of one goal may coincide with identification of a different goal. Moreover, science must be translated to affordable, acceptable, and accessible solutions to achieve broad effects, he contended.

Barriers to Personalized Nutrition Plan Uptake

Anthony noted that understanding and addressing individual lifestyle choices and behaviors are equally as important as biology. An Nlumn consumer study found that 57 percent of consumers are interested in personalized nutrition and health, and some consumers are already participating in a variety of ways, he reported. Out of 3,000 individuals interested in personalized and precision nutrition, 84 percent experimented with a different eating plan or style and 15 percent participated in personalized nutrition in the last year. More than 40 percent of participants regularly use digital apps to track health, and many are willing to share their data with companies that manage those apps. Consumers voiced that plentiful data are available to them, but making sense of data is challenging. Anthony noted that the COVID-19 pandemic affected many people's priorities; the most frequently reported consumer-desired benefits in the study included quality sleep, increased energy, general wellness, and mental and emotional health—participants ranked weight management and cardiovascular health as less important than these benefits. Anthony stated that research, anthropometrics, and biological markers are not yet robust enough for current consumer priorities; thus, he said, further efforts are needed to identify new markers and measure prioritized benefits.

Anthony highlighted that the value equation for personalized nutrition plans does not yet meet consumer needs, as the cost (measured in money and effort) is greater than the benefits. Indeed, the number one reason why people across all income groups cease using personalized nutrition plans is cost, he stated, adding that cost is the largest barrier to entry into using these plans, and many personalized nutrition plan users cease participation within 6 months. After cost, Anthony said, consumers most often cite lack of support as their reason for no longer participating in the plan. Although two-thirds of consumers seek a high level of support, only about one-third indicate they receive such support, he noted. Health care professionals are the most trusted source of desired support, yet most people receive support through online search engines, which often leads to feelings of frustration and being overwhelmed. Sectors can work together to deliver more effective personalized nutrition models, said Anthony. Academia can increase cross-disciplinary research, build diversity in datasets, and develop meaningful markers of health and disease, he asserted. Anthony stated that industry can make consumer behavior data accessible, support translation of data to behavior change and associated benefits, and deliver innovative solutions that support end benefits. And, he said, government can increase funding for health research, expand claim opportunities, and provide a structure for incentives for the democratization of personalized nutrition.

A Future Personalized Nutrition Scenario

Anthony described how personalized nutrition could soon look for consumers. In this example, a fictitious person, "Sara," recently lost 10 pounds and is pleased with her progress but struggles to reach her goal of losing 15 pounds before an upcoming reunion. Continuous sensors detect changes in satiety-related hormones, indicating a needed adjustment in energy and nutrients to support her goals and maintain body composition. Simultaneously, a hydration patch detects decreased hydration status during afternoons, which affects focus and contributes to hunger. In response to these data, Sara receives recommendations for afternoon beverages that meet her personal preferences as well as her biological needs. In addition, these data are communicated to her employer's smart beverage machine. Because the employer understands the value of productivity associated with a healthy workforce, the employer covers the cost of the beverages. Later, Sara invites her sister over for dinner. In preparation, her smart refrigerator recommends tweaks to favorite family dishes that align with her weight loss goals. The refrigerator produces a shopping list of ingredients. Technology enables Sara to partner with people seeking the same benefits in order to capitalize on volume discounts. Sara's weight loss reduces her risk calculation, and her health insurance company extends her a discount in response. She successfully reaches her goal weight and feels motivated to work toward a new goal of building the muscle needed to take up rock climbing. Anthony described this scenario as illustrating the cycle of benefits, measurement, information, and behavior change.

Anthony summarized that more tailored approaches to nutrition may be helpful in addressing chronic illness, reducing health care costs, and improving the health span. However, he said, demonstrating the efficacy of personalized nutrition plans is currently in the early stages. Consumers are seeking more personalized nutrition solutions, he continued, but a value gap between the price paid and the results received leads many individuals to stop participating in these programs within 6 months. Collaboration between sectors is needed to address the lack of alignment between science, consumer expectations, and outcomes to deliver evidence-based models that are accessible and affordable, said Anthony. Biomarkers related to chronic lifestyle diseases are heavily studied, and these diseases most often affect low-income and minoritized communities. Thereby, he said, personalized solutions hold potential to change the health trajectories of disenfranchised populations.

FOOD COMPOSITION AND THE
FUTURE OF NUTRITION AND HEALTH

Naomi K. Fukagawa, U.S. Department of Agriculture (USDA) Beltsville Human Nutrition Research Center, discussed USDA's efforts to provide data on food composition. For more than a century, the department has been responsible for monitoring food composition and intake. Its history of research in food composition, nutrition, and health began in the late 1800s and featured the work of Wilbur O. Atwater, who published *The Chemical Composition of American Food Materials* in 1906 (Atwater and Chas, 1896). In addition to monitoring food supply, intake, and dietary patterns, Fukagawa related, USDA provides food and nutrition data to researchers, policymakers, industry, health care providers, and consumers. She said the agency extends examination of food composition beyond nutrients to the discovery of new components and the identification of bioactive compounds that affect health and wellness. Research on the metabolic use of food components continues, and Fukagawa contended that this research must evolve in response to rapid changes in the food supply that occur with advances in science and technology. Numerous factors affect food composition, she said, including agricultural practices, analytical approaches, communication and data sharing, understanding of diet–disease interactions, climate change, and growing populations. These factors ultimately affect nutrition education and policy, Fukagawa pointed out.

The varied users of food composition information require a "modernized" approach to using the data provided by USDA FoodData Central, which Fukagawa described as an integrated data system launched by USDA in 2019 to provide expanded nutrient profile data and links to related agricultural and experimental research (Agricultural Research Service, 2019). She explained that the system features five distinct data types that are related but not necessarily interchangeable, including (1) Foundation Foods; (2) National Nutrient Database for Standard Reference Legacy 2018; (3) Food and Nutrient Database for Dietary Studies; (4) USDA Global

Branded Food Products database; and (5) Experimental Foods. Information within each data type is collected with unique acquisition approaches and for specific applications. USDA has prioritized efforts to manage high volumes of data to enable data science and personalized or precision nutrition, Fukagawa noted. The department is working to embody FAIR data principles—i.e., data that are findable, accessible, interoperable, and reusable—within a flexible database network (Wilkinson et al., 2016). *Findable* data contain unique identifiers for data systems. *Accessible* data are open and free for public use. *Interoperable* data can be used with other data and other vocabularies. *Reusable* data enable automated meta-analyses and study replication from similar studies. Effectively using data to enable precision or personalized nutrition involves melding systems biology with data science, she explained.

Fukagawa outlined challenges USDA faces in meeting current data needs. She asserted that dietary intake assessment must be revisited, noting that the Beltsville Human Nutrition Research Center Food Surveys Research Group is undertaking this effort as part of the National Health and Nutrition Examination Survey. USDA must prioritize the analysis of certain food components because analyzing all components is not feasible, she said, and greater understanding is needed of the bioavailability of food components, food interactions, and individual metabolism. Moreover, Fukagawa stated, these mechanisms are affected by factors—such as genetics, the environment, management procedures, and processing—that require deeper exploration within the context of planetary health. A future vision of an integrated food and health ecosystem should include food composition, she maintained, noting that it constitutes a gap in some models. For instance, a model of precision nutrition includes multiple omics (multiomics), lifestyle changes, demographics, habits, and physical activity, but omits food composition (USDA, 2019). Algorithms that predict the healthiest foods and food quantities for individual consumption should include compositional analysis with high-quality data, Fukagawa contended. A sustainable food system provides adequate nutritious foods for the growing population while also protecting the environment. Creating such a system will require understanding how to integrate sustainable production with nutrient optimization (i.e., food composition) and developing new paradigms for realizing sustainable food systems, she said.

Numerous long-term challenges related to food composition remain to be addressed in fostering a strong future for nutrition and health, said Fukagawa. Ensuring data quality is foremost among these challenges, she remarked, as the data need to be transparent, easily accessible, usable, and linkable. Fukagawa stated that multiomics related to food and health outcomes should be incorporated, and that marketing and profit considerations for producers, manufacturers, and consumers are at play. Efforts are needed to define wellness and establish biomarkers of food quality and health, she said. These challenges can be met through collaborative, cooperative dialogue and public–private partnerships, Fukagawa noted, highlighting the Food Forum as a vehicle for such collaboration. Furthermore, a balance in embracing tradition and new technologies can be achieved via workforce development, she said; a workforce capable of meeting current challenges will feature integrative physiologists, listeners, and communicators—given the general breakdown of clear communication in recent years—and transdisciplinary teams of scientists. Fukagawa stated that the diversity within collaborations should extend beyond disciplines to include different generations, bringing together forward thinking and expertise to solve the problems facing the food system. She emphasized that the focus should extend beyond single nutrients and single outcomes. Instead, she urged taking a systems approach to biology, food production, and ensuring the health of humans and the planet, in order to bridge the availability, accessibility, affordability, and acceptability of food.

FOOD AND NUTRITION SECURITY AND EQUITY

Angela Odoms-Young, Cornell University, described equity trends in the nutrition and health field and considerations for future security and equity. She said that, despite technological advances and the development of advanced data science techniques—including human genome sequencing—over the past 30 years, the high burden of chronic disease in the United States persists. In 2019, she reported, 53 percent of adults aged 18–34 years had at least one chronic condition, and 22 percent had multiple chronic conditions (Watson et al., 2019). She emphasized that the prevalence was higher in some population subgroups, with this high disease burden generating substantial economic and social costs. Odoms-Young said that issues of equity are evident in the higher rates of diet-related morbidity and mortality, maternal morbidity and mortality, and infant mortality experienced by specific subpopulations. Disparities related to race, socioeconomic status, health insurance coverage, geographical location, gender, sexuality, citizenship, disability, and age demonstrate that the disease burden disproportionately affects certain populations, she stated.

Odoms-Young discussed shifts within diet-related disease research and interventions over the past three decades. In the past, she explained, the primary focus was an individual's choice between healthy and unhealthy foods. She highlighted that research on drivers of health disparities focused on the role of culture, and interventions in the 1980s and 1990s incorporated this focus in teaching culturally appropriate dietary practices and cooking techniques. However, she said, research on social and structural determinants of health has become far more robust and demonstrates that individual, structural, and social levels all contribute to diet-related disease disparities. Upstream factors—including governance, socioeconomic position, education, social policies, and public policies—contribute to material, behavioral, biological, and psychosocial dynamics, Odoms-Young asserted, which in turn impact equity, health, and well-being, as well as social cohesion and social capital (Solar and Irwin, 2010). Health systems and other systems are drivers of health and affect individual health and dietary behaviors. Moreover, she said, structural oppression drives racial discrimination and disparities in housing and income, while the inequitable distribution of resources drives social conditions that create disparities in food and nutrition security. Odoms-Young cited a study that found the mean 10-year risk of cardiovascular disease, adjusted for age and sex, was significantly higher in non-Hispanic Black participants compared with White participants (He et al., 2015). Further adjustment for education, income, home ownership, health insurance and access to care, and employment attenuated the difference in health outcomes, she reported.

Odoms-Young outlined efforts needed to advance science to achieve improved dietary behaviors, nutrition outcomes, and health outcomes in terms of diet-related conditions. She explained that team science coalesces expertise from fields such as social science, AI, biological sciences, and genetics to consider the modification of various factors to improve health. Implementation science can increase the fidelity and effectiveness of interventions to change systems, she continued; it can also address drivers of poor diet and health outcomes at the programmatic, policy, and population levels. Furthermore, said Odoms-Young, the context of complex structural factors should be considered in downstream interventions such as precision nutrition. She stated that accelerated reduction of health disparities and improved diet and health outcomes require broader approaches that intervene in socioeconomic, environmental, and system-level factors. Odoms-Young asserted that structural, behavioral, and biomedical interventions are needed; that these should be rigorously evaluated and evidence based, she continued, and should address the social determinants of health that systematically lead to and perpetuate social and health inequities (Brown et al., 2019; Goldenberg et al., 2021).

Odoms-Young concluded by describing the concept of *Sankofa*. Originating with the Akan people of Ghana and embraced throughout the African Diaspora, Sankofa represents the idea that knowing the history and heritage of one's self and culture enables people to better themselves and their world. Applied to nutritional sciences, Odoms-Young explained, Sankofa can represent understanding historical and cultural factors to build on what has worked well and learn from what has not, such as policies that have generated societal inequities. Illustrating the intersection of structural factors, community resources, food access, and health, she gave the example of the Tops Friendly Markets supermarket in Buffalo, New York, where a mass shooting took place in 2022. This market offers increased access to food in the area and remains open for business. Odoms-Young pointed out that nutrition and food security exist in a broader context than individual choice alone, and social justice, food justice, food equity, and food sovereignty are components of potential solutions.

DISCUSSION

The discussion following the presentations summarized above focused on food insecurity among U.S. students; the evidence base for precision nutrition; and AI and diversity, equity, and inclusion (DEI) in the food system.

Food Insecurity Among U.S. Students

Ajay P. Malshe, Purdue University, asked about steps to address the high rates of food insecurity facing students. Odoms-Young replied that one of her undergraduate students completed a meta-synthesis on food insecurity among college students that revealed contributing factors and potential solutions. The review found that housing costs affect the income available for food, she said. College students who come from economically disadvantaged families are often in need of additional resources, continued Odoms-Young. She shared that several pilot projects have worked to address campus food needs, such as charitable food distribution via college-based food pantries and enrolling eligible students in food assistance programs. Potential structural solutions include colleges and universities subsidizing meal plans and housing costs for economically disadvantaged students, she remarked. Fukagawa noted that food insecurity affects communities throughout the United States and worldwide. Programs that reuse food waste in a safe manner are a potential solution for providing nutrition to all people in need. Malshe commented that packaged ramen noodles are a popular and inexpensive food choice among students, and the production of more nutritious ramen noodles could benefit this population.

Precision Nutrition Evidence Base

Peter Lurie, Center for Science in the Public Interest, remarked that precision nutrition proposals hold promise for reimagining nutrition service delivery in ways that may be complicated and expensive. He asked about evidence indicating that a precision nutrition approach can improve health outcomes. Anthony clarified that precision and personalized nutrition are different, with the former addressing specific dietary needs of a group of people with a common condition, such as type 2 diabetes or cardiovascular disease. For example, he said, research has explored the risk of cardiovascular disease and type 2 diabetes in relation to higher-fat versus lower-fat diets. Established markers related to disease can be combined with methodologies for understanding the differences between individuals to target specific dietary recommendations, he said, noting that food companies can support precision nutrition without conducting single-subject studies. As an example, Anthony said that companies can improve the nutritional quality of their products consistent with their consumers' dietary needs. He added that technology is not yet able to robustly deliver personalized nutrition at the individual level.

Fukagawa remarked that the goal of precision nutrition is understanding how the components of various foods may enhance wellness. Current basic understanding is that humans need adequate food—not too little or too much—and diversity in food intake, she said. People with specific medical conditions, such as metabolic disorders, may benefit from a truly specialized diet, she continued, but a specific prescribed diet for optimal health has not been established for the general population. Lurie replied that specific diets for people with metabolic disorders constitute treatment for a clinical condition. He clarified that Anthony is referring to a wholly different approach to public health nutrition that does away with broad recommendations and instead makes specific, individualized recommendations. Before making such a dramatic change, evidence that this new approach will improve health should be in place, Lurie maintained. In clinical medicine, practitioners prescribe medications that are likely to treat patients' medical conditions effectively and avoid prescribing medications likely to cause adverse effects in certain individuals, he noted. He then asked about the status of the field of personalized nutrition in terms of being capable of similarly recommending intake or avoidance of specific foods. Anthony stated that a few studies have examined the benefits of individualized diets versus general dietary guidance, but the evidence base is still developing. He remarked that widespread guidance, such as reducing sodium intake, is helpful and is supported by data, but dietary guidance does not necessarily address behavior. Anthony contended that personalized approaches may influence behavior more effectively by connecting recommendations to specific needs or goals. Whereas general guidance tells people what to do, he explained, precision nutrition addresses individual needs and offers recommendations that are consistent with a person's needs, culture, and preferences. Furthermore, precision nutrition is not limited to medical needs or food as medicine; it extends to individual needs and goals that may not be related to medical conditions.

Artificial Intelligence and Diversity, Equity, and Inclusion in the Food System

Christina Chauvenet, Newman's Own Foundation, asked about the opportunities and challenges associated with AI in the food system in terms of health equity and nutrition, noting that AI sometimes perpetuates biases. Odoms-Young acknowledged issues of bias within data and algorithms that train AI across fields. Data science groups are working to address these issues, she said, but much work remains to be done in this area. Some companies are exploring the intersection of AI and DEI with a specific focus on using AI to address social inequities, she noted. And she pointed out that developing the capability to adjust inputs in terms of differences in housing, income, and other social and structural determinants of health holds promise in using AI to achieve the best outcomes possible. The nutrition space often focuses on a physiological or biological focus; broadening this to include biological inputs and omics with social and structural determinants of health could yield a better understanding of how to address inequities, said Odoms-Young. She noted that evidence on the effectiveness of DEI approaches indicates that DEI works by informing the types of questions scientists ask and the methods they apply. For instance, she said, researchers should consider social and structural determinants of health in community nutrition, and DEI efforts in the field of nutrition could also support diverse training and practitioners. She added that the registered dietitian workforce is not currently representative of the populations bearing higher disease burden, such as racial minority groups, disability communities, and LGBTQ+ communities.

Khoo asked about the use of technology to increase knowledge of food composition and address needs within population subgroups. Fukagawa stated that these efforts begin with high-quality data, which can be expensive and challenging to collect, especially given that new compounds appear in food that have claims of related positive physiological outcomes. Once sufficient quality data are achieved, she noted, AI can be used to help identify solutions. Multiple factors and nonlinear relationships are likely at play in terms of the effects of food composition on health outcomes, she said, adding that partnerships and data sharing between industry and academia are mechanisms for collecting adequate quality data. Fukagawa emphasized that food is not a pharmaceutical, food is a necessity. As people eat throughout their lifetimes, their bodies respond to different foods in various ways depending on environment, genetics, and various other factors, she said. Food cannot be regulated or prescribed in the same way that pharmaceuticals are, she explained, as the former is imperative and the latter optional. Fukagawa shared that she uses the acronym "DEIA" in reference to foods to recommend that one's plate should feature *diversity* of foods, *equity* across food groups with no one group overrepresented, *inclusivity* by using multiple foods and approaches to cooking, and being *affordable* and *accessible*.

6

A Visionary Perspective on
the Future of Food

The fifth session of the symposium featured a presentation on a vision for the future of food that explored the effects of the food system on health, the environment, and socioeconomics; provided an overview of the *National Food Strategy* in the United Kingdom; and outlined efforts to support transformation of the food system toward sustainability and human and planetary health. Guy Poppy, UK Research and Innovation (UKRI), described how regional, national, and local systems operate within the global food system, noting that some policy and fiscal levers can be used to initiate change at the local and national levels that are not at play at the global level. UKRI is an overarching body of a series of research councils and the largest public funder of research and innovation in the United Kingdom, investing £8 billion annually in research efforts. The organization brings together scientists from a variety of fields; those relevant to the food system include engineering, medicine, economics, social sciences, and biotechnology and biological sciences.

FOOD SYSTEM EFFECTS ON HEALTH AND ENVIRONMENT

Poppy stated that a vision for a future food system is needed to address harmful consequences of the current food system on the planet and on general health. Although food system development has successfully met post–World War II caloric needs of the general population, it has done so at a cost to human and environmental health, he explained. More than 820 million people around the world are undernourished, he reported, and approximately 2 billion people face moderate or severe food

47

insecurity in relation to micronutrient deficiency or shortages in calories at certain periods of time. Simultaneously, approximately 2 billion adults and 380 million children have obesity or overweight, he said; rising rates of obesity worldwide increase risks for type 2 diabetes, cardiovascular disease, and cancer. Prior to the COVID-19 pandemic, noncommunicable diseases had a greater effect on death rates than communicable disease, Poppy continued. He noted that susceptibility to COVID-19 infection and related consequences of infection proved to be higher for people with obesity and/or who have certain diseases associated with obesity. In terms of environmental effects, Poppy said, the food system contributes one-third of emitted greenhouse gases, uses half of global habitable land, requires 70 percent of global freshwater use, and contributes 78 percent of eutrophication pollution to oceans and fresh water (Ritchie et al., 2022). Furthermore, he stated, livestock constitute 94 percent of global mammal biomass. Given these effects within the context of a changing climate and growing populations, Poppy urged, future human and planetary health calls for a new food system.

Poppy described global food system challenges. During a large U.K. research program running since 2019, he said, dramatic shifts in climate change and associated extreme weather events have occurred, making the research even more important. A move toward net-zero greenhouse gas emissions will require significant change within the food system to be successful. Poppy emphasized that agriculture should be part of the solution for achieving net-zero greenhouse gas emissions, rather than a part of the problem. Agricultural land use and associated loss of biodiversity and soil health pose risks to future harvests, he said, especially where land is subjected to the effects of climate change. Food security faces challenges from a growing population and shocks to the food supply. He underscored the extent to which global challenges related to nutrition, food safety, and social inequalities pose risks to human health and place further strain on a food system that is already overburdened.

NATIONAL FOOD STRATEGY

Poppy explained that a food systems approach considers the food supply chain within a complex context of political, health, environmental, societal, and economic systems. Within this interconnected network, he said, a focus narrowed to any one system can lead to unintended consequences in other systems (Parsons et al., 2019). Thus, a systems approach aids in avoiding harmful effects by identifying connections between systems, stated Poppy. Commissioned by the U.K. government, the 2021 *National Food Strategy* is the first independent review of England's food system in

75 years (UKRI, 2023).[1] The review lays out a vision and plan for a better food system and includes 14 recommendations based within four central themes, Poppy stated. The first theme is escaping the "junk food cycle" and protecting the National Health Service (NHS) from the costs of diet-related health conditions associated with the current food system. Poppy noted that during the COVID-19 pandemic, the phrase "protect the NHS" became part of public health efforts encouraging people to modify their behavior. The second and third themes are reducing diet-related inequality and making the best use of land. Given that land is a limited resource and the population is growing, he explained, multiple needs for land will inevitably compete with one another. The last theme is creating a long-term shift in food culture, one that transforms the food system into a new state.

TRANSFORMING U.K. FOOD SYSTEMS

Poppy described how the Transforming U.K. Food Systems Strategic Priorities Fund—a partnership between UKRI and several governmental departments—aims to fundamentally transform the U.K. food system by centering healthy people and a healthy natural environment. He said the research program focuses on the United Kingdom while recognizing the global context of the food system. Dedicating £47.5 million to research efforts, the program will publish findings from funded projects as well as a blueprint for transforming the U.K. food system in an anticipated 2025 volume from the scientific journal *Philosophical Transactions of the Royal Society*. Poppy outlined the program's goals:

1. transforming U.K. diets to be healthier and more sustainable;
2. changing the behavior of actors across the food system;
3. modeling interdependencies throughout the food system;
4. coproducing research between academia and stakeholders from national and local government, the private sector, and civil society organizations; and
5. developing a pipeline of skilled people able to apply critical interdisciplinary systems thinking to the food system.

He underscored the importance of coproduced research in achieving translation and intended effects within the food system. The workforce pipeline aims to produce 60 doctoral students trained in food systems thinking whose Ph.D. work focuses on the U.K. food system. He stated his hope that these students would go on to work within the food system,

---

[1] Poppy acknowledged that although it is described as "national," the strategy applies only to England and does not include Scotland, Wales, or Northern Ireland.

rather than in academia, to achieve the greatest possible effect on the food system.

Poppy noted the activities of the Transforming U.K. Food Systems program to date, such as establishment of the Center for Doctoral Training. Four large consortia with 5-year timelines and 12 smaller 2- to 3-year research projects are underway. Poppy described how the program has published several reports, including a study on mapping the U.K. food system that demonstrates the complexity of a network that contains approximately 600,000 food businesses. Another report explores the levers for food system transformation and discusses policies and efforts that have been successful within the United Kingdom or in other nations. And a report on public procurement of food examines the role of schools, hospitals, and other public service organizations in providing food within communities. In some cities, Poppy stated, more than half of all food is publicly procured, demonstrating an opportunity to make progress toward sustainability and health through school and hospital leadership. The program is supporting projects across the United Kingdom on issues including trade, food waste, eating practices, and food service, he said. And he added that the information generated by these projects is already being used to shape policy and exert influence on various parts of the food system.

Poppy described various Transforming U.K. Food Systems projects that are currently underway. A project based at Reading University—which relates to the *National Food Strategy* theme of escaping the junk food cycle and protecting the NHS—is exploring the use of fruit and vegetable incentivization in disadvantaged communities to improve access to and availability of produce. Poppy explained that increasing fiber and micronutrient intake within these communities can have effects on public health. However, he said, messaging on incorporating fruits and vegetables into diet does not necessarily translate to behavior change and health gains. Two projects aimed at reducing diet-related inequality use "health by stealth" methods of increasing the nutrient content in white bread, with one project using pulses and the other using higher-fiber wheat. Incorporating these products into the bread supply chain does not require a change in business model or in consumer preferences, as the shift in ingredients does not affect the taste of the bread, Poppy reported. He stated that two slices of modified bread can provide 40 percent of recommended daily fiber intake to a portion of the population consuming very little fiber and not responding to messaging about fruit and vegetable intake. White bread is widely consumed by this subpopulation; thus, he said, a modified product offers potential improvement in health. Poppy noted that these projects involve working with manufacturers, retailers, and consumer panels. Related to the theme of making best use of land, another project is developing bean seed, designed to thrive in the United Kingdom, that can be incorporated into processed foods, ready-meals, and school lunches. And a project working toward the goal of creating a long-term shift in food culture is working with the city of Sheffield to incorporate aspects of public health, circular economy, and sustainability into a food plan, which in turn will inform food plans in cities across the United Kingdom. Poppy said that this effort involves procurement, advocacy, and health messaging.

INVESTING IN THE FUTURE OF FOOD

Poppy stated that UKRI spent £1.3 billion from 2016 to 2021 on food-related research and innovation. He led a UKRI Food Deep Dive to explore the organization's role in supporting the food system, which found that investment was overly siloed in directing funding toward projects focused on single areas, such as food production, diet research, or food manufacturing. Given that food system transformation will involve multidisciplinary efforts, he said, research projects should be collaborative and consider various areas of the food system (UKRI, 2023), and even a small project conducted by agricultural scientists can consider how this work applies within the broader food system. Poppy noted that he is currently in discussions with the U.K. government regarding efforts to address obesity and about the future formulation of foods in the context of concerns about ultra-processed foods. Investing in partnerships, he continued, UKRI supports strategic research programs and infrastructure such as the U.K. Food Safety Network and the Biofortification Hub. He stated that UKRI's international partnerships include the International Wheat Yield Partnership, which is working to increase the yield of wheat—the largest global source of calories—by 50 percent by 2035. And, he said, another project invests in venture capital–funded companies and small and midsize enterprises, which are often highly innovative in driving new ideas forward.

EXAMPLES OF FOOD SYSTEM SOLUTIONS

Poppy outlined various solutions to address issues related to health, the environment, and social economics, emphasizing that every initiative should be based in systems thinking. He said that Cathie Martin at the John Innes Centre has led research using gene editing and CRISPR-Cas9 on tomatoes, which she targeted because of their popularity among consumers and inclusion in a variety of food products (Li et al., 2022). Lack of sunlight contributes to a widespread vitamin D shortage in the United Kingdom that affects approximately one-third of the population during winter months, Poppy explained. Gene editing manipulates the enzyme that converts provitamin 3 to cholesterol, he said, which leads to an accumulation of vitamin D in the edited tomatoes. This effort builds on extensive work by

Martin's team to manipulate the nutritional composition of tomatoes and provides an example of how gene editing can target nutrition in well-liked products. Poppy remarked that many people find it difficult to eat five fruits or vegetables a day, and the goal of eating two nutrient-dense fruits or vegetables each day would be easier to achieve.

Poppy described the obesity crisis, which is growing in the United Kingdom and worldwide. The United Kingdom's treasury has expressed concerns about the effects of obesity on employee productivity and unemployment, he said. Current trends suggest that 51 percent of the global population will have overweight or obesity in 2035, Poppy reported, carrying an annual economic impact of more than $4 trillion, a sum comparable to the impact of COVID-19 in 2020 (World Obesity Federation, 2023). In the United Kingdom, NHS has begun prescribing glucagon-like peptide 1 (GLP-1) agonists to people with type 2 diabetes and high body mass index. Poppy surmised that for a small subset of people, GLP-1 agonists will be very advantageous, but these drugs alone will not solve the obesity crisis, and other solutions are needed.

Poppy discussed concerns related to ultra-processed foods, a topic that is frequently covered by the media. While some nutrition proponents argue that people should cook with fresh ingredients, he said, public surveys indicate that many people want to maintain the convenience of the current food system. Therefore, Poppy stated, changing the ways the foods are produced or formulated may be an avenue for providing foods that consumers want while reducing the risk of negative health effects associated with ultra-processed food intake. He said that shifting processing methods and ingredient contents while maintaining fibers that are important for gut microbiomes could potentially offer convenience and nutrition simultaneously. Poppy stated that more research is needed to understand whether the negative health effects seen with consumption of ultra-processed foods are caused by (1) the processing itself; (2) the content of ultra-processed foods, such as high levels of fat or sugar or the inclusion of other ingredients; or (3) a combination of processing and ingredients.

Poppy remarked on the use of innovation to meet environmental challenges associated with food production. Although fertilizers are important to current methods of food production, the Haber-Bosch process of creating fertilizers is highly energy intensive, he said. When an energy crisis rendered the Haber-Bosch process economically unfeasible, levels of carbon dioxide—a byproduct of Haber-Bosch—became so low in the United Kingdom that the food industry had no access to carbon dioxide, explained Poppy. He said that CCm Technologies has begun producing new low-carbon fertilizers by converting carbon captured from agricultural and industrial waste streams. Shown to be effective in a range of farming environments, these fertilizers are sold out until 2026. To demonstrate the high demand, Poppy noted that a company that purchased low-carbon fertilizers from CCm Technologies has offered to build an additional manufacturing plant in exchange for access to the product. These developments exemplify how innovation can provide access to desired products while decreasing or eliminating the associated harmful effects, he said. Poppy stated that the Green Revolution tripled cereal yield, enabling food production to meet the needs of a growing population without drastically increasing land use (Ritchie and Roser, 2019). He also noted that additional research could enable regenerative agriculture practices to maintain needed yield while reducing negative effects to the environment.

Poppy explored socioeconomic aspects of global trading within the food system, noting that the United Kingdom is a net importer of food. When factoring in costs associated with public health and the environment, he said, some food products cost almost twice as much as the price charged to consumers. However, if the full economic cost is applied to product price, this change would likely be most burdensome to people who can least afford to change their diet, he contended. Additionally, the world is producing a food supply that is misaligned with most dietary guidelines, such as those in the EAT-*Lancet* report or in the U.K. *Eatwell Guide*, said Poppy. This raises the question of how to encourage manufacturers, retailers, and consumers to modify diets to align food supply and demand with human and planetary health, he said. Poppy related that, in November 2023, Juergen Voegele, vice president for sustainable development at World Bank, contended that increased funding is not necessarily required to promote transformation. Voegele cited the $800 billion spent annually by governments worldwide on food production incentives that have negative effects on climate and environmental outcomes. Poppy remarked that government subsidies could shift to incentivize a new food system that supports human and planetary health.

Whereas other sectors—such as energy, aerospace, and car industries—each have a clear, shared vision for increasing sustainability and a plan for delivery, the food sector has not developed a shared vision, said Poppy. Scientists often disagree about the direction needed within the food sector, he said, thereby generating confusion among the public. Poppy stated that a variety of ideas on how to arrive at or contribute to a determined endpoint is healthy; however, the lack of a shared vision to work toward inhibits the ability to develop plans of delivery. Furthermore, he asserted, without a collective vision, articulating needed actions for world leaders and the public becomes difficult, thereby limiting collaboration.

7

Fireside Chat:
Food for Thought on the Next 30 Years

The sixth session of the symposium featured a discussion that spanned a range of topics, including technologies that could have substantial effects on the future food system; contextual challenges facing the food system; visions for the next 30 years of food system progress; issues related to health span, nutrition, and behavior change; consumer and industry responsibility for behavior change; consideration of Native American agricultural practices; and the role of the wealthiest individuals in change efforts. The session was moderated by Rodolphe Barrangou, North Carolina State University.

TECHNOLOGIES FOR THE FUTURE OF FOOD

Barrangou opened the discussion by highlighting the diversity of expertise among symposium participants, who represented academia, government, nongovernmental organizations, regulatory bodies, industry, and consumer groups. Underscoring the unprecedented pace and scale at which the world is changing, he asked about technologies that offer promise in contending with current and emerging challenges. Lauren Abda, Branchfood and Branch Venture Group (BVG), stated that BVG invests in food innovation businesses at the earliest phases of development. In exploring consumer product brands, food technology, and agriculture technology, Abda said, the investment group engages with scientists to understand the products they are bringing to market and how these products can be applied to improving the food system. She listed a wide range of innovations with food system applications: (1) technology to recreate animal-based products with plant-based ingredients; (2) technology that influences delivery; (3) technology involving sensors, drones, and robotics; (4) food manufacturing technology; and (5) pest-identification technology. Abda said that BVG strives to understand specific challenges within the food industry and identify how technology can be applied to add value and to support evolution toward sustainability, environmental friendliness, and better health outcomes. She contended that artificial intelligence (AI) will be the leading technology influencing the food system, as AI affects every point in the supply chain. Consumers use AI through search engines to obtain information about food options, she pointed out. For instance, people search for answers to questions such as, "I am dehydrated; what should I drink?" In response, she said, the search engine might issue an AI-generated reply about water and electrolyte-based beverages. At the farm level, AI will play a role in determining which genetic traits to include in seeds to develop plants that withstand environmental change and enhance human nutrition, said Abda.

Ajay P. Malshe, Purdue University, highlighted the deeply personal experiences that people have with food, as exhibited in the comfort and memories often associated with food. He added that referring to food as medicine does not capture the personal space that food occupies. Malshe maintained that agriculture and the food supply chain should be secure, trusted, and resilient. The potential effects of misinformation and rapid changes—including geopolitical events—pose challenges to the food system's security, credibility, and resilience, he observed. In the future, Malshe added, technologies will be needed that enable food production to be decoupled from water and land as much as possible. He reported that in the United States around 70–80 percent of the population lives in urban areas, yet only about 20 percent of food is produced in or near these locations. As the population continues to grow, Malshe continued, technologies that enable urban food production (e.g., urban farming, cellular agriculture) will be increasingly important to deliver food at points of need. He noted that cellular agriculture produces food through bioreactors and can be used to create new forms of protein that could complement current protein sources in the future.

Susan T. Mayne, former director of the Center for Food Safety and Applied Nutrition at the U.S. Food and Drug Administration, emphasized the potential of gene editing to address numerous challenges related to the food system. Crops can be genetically engineered or gene edited to be more resistant to effects of climate change, such as drought, she said. Moreover, the nutritional quality of food can be enhanced through gene editing. Food waste, which contributes to greenhouse gas emissions, could be reduced by protecting crops from emerging pathogens, thereby simultaneously shielding farmers from economic losses, she asserted. Despite the benefits gene editing offers, scientific misinformation and consumer lack of understanding pose challenges to its application, Mayne continued. As demonstrated by the public response to genetically modified organisms, she said, efforts are needed to improve science communications through social media and other avenues. Gene editing—and its potential to address climate change, food waste, and nutrition needs—should be supported through effective communication efforts.

Xavier Morales, The Praxis Project, described how his organization collaborates with power-building groups nationwide that are working to transform systems, structures, and policies that underlie inequity or injustice. Food is a major area of injustice, he stated, as evidenced by the one-third of students experiencing food insecurity and the increasing demand for food bank services. Ironically, amid enormous amounts of food waste, people in the United States are going hungry. Thus, in addition to advancing technologies, parallel efforts should explore food inequities and develop a vision for the food system, he contended. Whether the vision is healthier people or food security for all, Morales continued, a vision could serve to center focus and efforts. He noted that the concept of *Sankofa*—looking to the past in order to move forward—can guide problem-solving by examining what has worked in the past that can be built upon and scaled.

Guy Poppy, UK Research and Innovation (UKRI), remarked that technology alone will not solve all of the issues facing the food system. He commented that data sharing involving both government departments and the private sector could be helpful in addressing these challenges. Achieving a large data signal enables early action and informs decision making. For example, he said, creation of digital twins (i.e., virtual models) supports real-time response to events. He noted that a large company based in Switzerland has more data about foods than do most government departments, indicating the potential value of data sharing. The combination of big data and AI holds potential for revolutionizing many aspects of the food system, Poppy maintained. Barrangou observed that all panelists noted a role for science and technology in creating solutions to food system challenges, and that Morales emphasized the importance of context in problem-solving.

CONTEXTUAL FOOD SYSTEM CHALLENGES

Barrangou highlighted contextual challenges facing the food system, including issues related to diversity, equity, and inclusion; access; affordability; trust; acceptance; communication; disinformation and misinformation; climate change; workforce training, acquisition, and retention; globalization; the global supply chain; and geopolitical forces. He asked about contextual challenges creating the greatest impediments to food system advancement. Morales replied that profit-seeking within a commercialized food system leads to inefficiencies within communities. Efforts to optimize health and nutrition are not always inclusive, and many Americans contend with hunger and inadequate access to food, he said. Morales noted that the COVID-19 pandemic demonstrated inequities within the food system. He highlighted a pandemic-response program implemented in Zuni Pueblo, New Mexico, in which rain barrels and home garden supplies were distributed to all residents, enabling them to grow their own food during a period of food system disruption. Optimization should seek benefits for all people rather than financial profits, he maintained. Morales described his advocacy efforts to bring health and science data to the attention of legislators and regulators in order to change policy; powerful economic interests often oppose these efforts, and Morales noted that his organization loses far more battles for equitable policies than it wins.

Mayne emphasized the need to address social determinants of health, such as poverty, in ameliorating food system challenges. Obesity often starts in childhood and thus requires a focus on food and nutrition for young people, she asserted. Currently approved medical treatments, including glucagon-like peptide 1 (GLP-1) agonists, are not approved or targeted for younger children, a time at which obesity often begins, Mayne noted; what is more, she said, GLP-1 is not effective for all consumers in older age groups, which underscores the need to address social determinants of health. Mayne added that misinformation amplified by social media undermines all goals for the food system. For consumers to demand healthier foods and thereby affect market forces—which, in turn, would lead to shifts in food production—consumers need accurate information, she said.

Malshe discussed the effects of human behavior in the context of food system challenges. As an immigrant to the United States, he expressed his perplexity at the common practice of drinking iced beverages throughout the winter. Ice production requires energy, a process that emits carbon, and much ice is discarded. Yet, this common practice is not discussed in addressing climate change, he stated. Additionally, human behavior is demonstrated in the choice to eat out in restaurants, which could be related to the perception that eating out reflects a good quality of life, Malshe contended. Providing contrast, he recounted growing up in a frugal household in which delicious, nutritious food was prepared daily and eating at a restaurant was viewed as lavish. Furthermore, despite the large percentages of Americans experiencing food insecurity and the common experience of seeing unhoused people, he asserted, most people in the United States do not accept that the nation faces a hunger challenge. Malshe stated that these examples reflect the role of human behavior in practices and perceptions related to food.

Abda remarked that in determining its investments, BVG considers value creation not only in terms of generating profit, but also in the value brought to people and society, including health and local economies. For example, Ocean Approved, a BVG portfolio company, has a consumer product brand, Atlantic Sea Farms, that sells seaweed food products. Based in Maine, the company grows seaweed in the ocean during wintertime, harvests in April, and blanches and processes the seaweed to create consumer products. Given that seaweed is a carbon sequestering sea vegetable, Abda noted, farming seaweed offers benefits to the environment. Moreover, seaweed is rich in iodine, a mineral that has decreased in some diets with the rise in popularity of non-iodized sea salt. Abda emphasized that when consumption of fortified products declines, it becomes important to identify replacement sources of nutrients. Atlantic Sea Farms also provides employment opportunities to the Maine lobstering community, which has been affected by the climate change–related migration of lobster further north, Abda explained. The company employs lobstermen and fishermen to plant kelp in the water through fishing lines inoculated with selected kelp seed spores and to harvest the kelp. Thus, the community retains jobs and continues to use materials and infrastructure developed in the area. This example illustrates how value creation extends beyond financial gains to offer benefit to the environment, health, and community, Abda added.

Poppy remarked that food waste is a pressing contextual concern. Various negative effects are associated with food production, and yet 30–40 percent of the food supply produced is discarded. He surmised that any other industry, such as the auto or pharmaceutical industry, would respond to that level of waste with prompt action to determine solutions. He added that in November 2023, King Charles III launched the Coronation Food Project, which is aimed at reducing food waste and hunger simultaneously by redistributing surplus food to food charities and community groups.

VISION FOR FOOD SYSTEM PROGRESS

Barrangou invited the panelists to imagine the Food Forum's 60th anniversary and to anticipate what topics and accomplishments will emerge in the interim. Abda commented on the high level of system coordination that will be required to achieve substantial accomplishments within the interconnected food system. Technology offers new possibilities, but an innovation will be adopted only if industry sees potential value in its application, she stated. It will be necessary to adopt technology at scale to create value for consumers in terms of health, efficiency, and systems optimization; this scaling will require system coordination. Abda continued that technology integration is a challenge that calls for a willingness to initiate and navigate change, which can be fostered through incentivization and funding. The pressing need to ameliorate climate change calls for the prioritization of efforts to coordinate the system and usher in solutions, Abda contended. She stated her hope that a collective mindset focused on the benefit of key players across the food value chain will yield substantial accomplishments over the next three decades.

Malshe echoed the need for integration, specifying that horizontal integration—across physical technology and platforms, digital operations and system interoperability, and sustainability—should be coupled with vertical integration of micronutrients. He emphasized that innovative physical technology often requires a minimum of 8 years to move from ideation to a realized commercial launch platform. In contrast, the hunt for digital technology "unicorns" (i.e., startup companies that achieve valuation of $1 billion) shortens the time allocated to developing a new digital technology idea to approximately 2 years, said Malshe. Thus, digital technology is more likely than physical technology to accelerate transformation. He predicted that a focus on sustainability will become more widespread with the increasing influence of the younger generation, which is accustomed to climate change and war. Malshe stated that value does not need to be created, because value already exists within the younger generation, and this generation will catalyze transformation.

Mayne shared a vision for 30 years hence in which market forces change the food system. Currently, food companies produce food that meets consumer demands and is profitable. Therefore, creating demand for nutritious, healthy, safe foods would exert market force on companies, she maintained. Industry, government, consumer groups, researchers, and academics could collaborate holistically to identify a path in generating market forces. In September 2022, the White House released *The National Strategy on Hunger, Nutrition, and Health*, which outlines U.S. initiatives to change the food system. Mayne underscored that subsidies could be better leveraged in driving market forces to a healthy, nutritious, and safe food supply.

Morales asserted that in 30 years, people will likely realize that efforts to solve a social problem through science and technology is too narrowly focused. Economic power and systems mapping tools should be considered during the exploration of why some people do not have enough food in an advanced technological society, he stated. Subsidies are an important lever, but despite the common knowledge that fruits and vegetables are healthy, the majority of U.S. subsidies support commodities that are not as healthy, said Morales. For instance, he noted, an article by Tillotson (2004) indicated that consumption of subsidized commodities increases rates of metabolic syndrome, heart disease, and stroke. Support is needed for policies and subsidies that align with recommended dietary guidelines. Morales described his vision for the next three decades as including the collective realization that technological solutions do not solve social problems, a shift to cooperative problem-solving, and a shared goal of eradicating hunger for all.

Poppy's vision of progress for the next 30 years features a 50 percent decrease in food waste and substantial movement toward diets that support the planet while maintaining health. He recounted speaking at an art school and encouraging the artists to use their mediums to convey powerful messages about needed change. Stating his optimism for the future, Poppy characterized Generation Z as agents of change, noting that some young people in the United Kingdom are radically changing their diets through conversion to veganism. He underscored the importance of ensuring adequate nutrition, such as sufficient intake of B vitamins, when changing diet. Some young people view health issues as concerns for their parents' and grandparents' generations, but decisions made during youth can affect long-term health. Poppy highlighted a need to support members of the younger generation both in their push for change and in maintaining their health; doing so will enable them to convert more and more people to diets that are healthy for humans and for the environment.

HEALTH SPAN, NUTRITION, AND BEHAVIOR CHANGE

Naomi K. Fukagawa, U.S. Department of Agriculture (USDA) Beltsville Human Nutrition Research Center, recounted technology advances 30 years ago, during her time as a pediatric resident, that enabled most sick infants and children to be kept alive. However, she said, the process of adopting this technology did not consider the various effects of extensive intervention to extend life on pediatric patients and their families. She asked how technology and interventions in the food space can be balanced with the associated effects on people and on the planet to avoid unintended consequences of technological advances. For example, she wondered whether foods modified to have increased vitamin content could have unintended health consequences for certain populations.

Poppy referred to the Malthusian principle, which assumes that when population growth exceeds the rate of increase in food supply, it results in catastrophe (e.g., war, famine, natural disasters). Thus, it could be argued that technology to temporarily increase food supply could result in an even larger number of people facing eventual catastrophe. He cited the *Chief Medical Officer's Annual Report 2023*, in which Chris Whitty, England's chief medical officer, emphasized that medical interventions during youth and later in life have succeeded in extending longevity, but the health span has not seen proportionate increases in length. As a result, the duration of chronic illness in older age, which is often diet related, has increased in length. Poppy noted that many people have described the National Health Service as a "national treatment service" that provides medical interventions but does not provide services, such as dietary interventions, to keep people healthy. Instead, funding is funneled toward medical treatment and secondary medical care.

Poppy remarked that a carrying capacity is at play, and that perhaps a focus on interventions to extend life should shift to interventions that improve long-term health and reduce the gap between longevity and healthy lifespan. Barrangou commented on the unique potential of nutrition and healthy foods to prevent the onset of disease and suggested that investing resources toward prevention efforts could yield greater benefit than investment in curing disease. Compelling people to ask for healthy foods would lead to production of healthy foods, which in turn could decrease disease and improve the health span, he maintained. Morales cautioned that a calculation of carrying capacity is contingent on societal factors. For instance, he said, the carrying capacity of a world full of people from the United States could be different than a world populated with people from Costa Rica.

Regarding behavior change as a disease-prevention mechanism, Morales emphasized that efforts to educate consumers about healthier options and to ensure those foods are available are at odds with strong industry forces that digitally market to children and promote unhealthy products through placement, pricing, and promotion. He gave the example of communities in California where soda is less expensive than water. He recalled that actress Jennifer Garner raised awareness about food deserts on a *Today Show* interview that featured a tour of Alpaugh, California. Ironically, the area surrounding this farming community grows half of the nation's produce, yet Alpaugh's lone grocery store does not carry a single fruit or vegetable. The focus on behavior change often overlooks environmental factors that do not support desired behaviors, said Morales. He proposed that efforts to change corporate behavior in terms of product promotion, pricing, and placement should accompany efforts to influence individual behavior.

CONSUMER AND INDUSTRY RESPONSIBILITY

Christian Peters, USDA Agricultural Research Service, asked about the responsibility of the consumer vis-à-vis the responsibility of the other components of the food system. Abda replied that many consumers want the food industry to offer healthier products featuring fewer ingredients that are natural, organic, and/or regenerative. The book *The Omnivore's Dilemma* and documentary *Seaspiracy* reflect discourse on concerns about the food industry. Consumers want options they feel they are not getting, she stated. Furthermore, Abda continued, despite the Hispanic population being the fastest-growing portion of the U.S. population, mass retailers offer few Hispanic-originated foods. As an example, she described five stores that sell baked goods near her office in Boston—none of them carry concha, a traditional Mexican sweet roll, despite the substantial number of Hispanic employees who work in her building. The products that the

U.S. food industry produces and distributes domestically do not reflect the diversity of the U.S. population, said Abda. At the same time, she asserted, consumer demand is driving companies to bring more foods to market that have better effects on health and the environment, demonstrating the power of the consumer voice. Be that as it may, industry has more work ahead in meeting consumer demand, Abda contended.

Poppy remarked on the concept of "food citizenship." The understanding that food choices affect climate and the environment leads some people to change their diets. He contended that self-identification as a "food citizen" could spur more rapid behavior change than identification as a consumer. Morales maintained that discussions of consumer responsibility must consider that consumers are diverse in their perspectives, economic power, agency, and access to healthy food. Some people living in communities where healthy foods are not readily available strive to eat the healthiest diet they can access within their environment. He recounted that during a conference presentation, a behavioral psychologist explained that people experiencing high levels of stress may begin their day with resolve to eat and drink healthy food, but mounting pressures throughout the day can erode that resolve. Thereby, a person's level of agency and the extent to which they consider the health aspects of foods can vary across the day. Morales cautioned against a narrow focus on consumer responsibility and called for efforts to address social determinants of health and corporate responsibility.

NATIVE AMERICAN FOOD SYSTEMS

Christina Chauvenet, Newman's Own Foundation, described Native American food systems as situated at the intersection of human health and environmental stewardship. Given the influence of subsidies and corporate profit on the foods available, she asked how Native American voices can be amplified to apply Native knowledge to problem-solving efforts. Malshe noted collaboration between Purdue University and Navajo nations on agriculture and food programs. The nexus of technology and food involves a social angle, he remarked. Food carries connections to history, traditions, cultures, and beliefs. Whereas technology changes quickly through the rapid launch of new products, upgrades, and software, many people continue to eat in adulthood the foods that they ate in childhood, said Malshe. Additionally, he said, the implementation of technologies that depend on natural resources face setting-specific challenges, such as water shortages in New Mexico and associated radioactive ground contamination. This raises the question of whether technologies can assist in decoupling dependency on natural resources, Malshe remarked.

ROLE OF THE WEALTHY IN CHANGE EFFORTS

A participant emphasized that not all consumers are created equal: a small minority of people have disproportionate levels of wealth and consumption of resources, thereby generating the largest carbon footprint. Despite the shifts in behaviors and attitudes evident in Generation Z, young people continue to idolize rich celebrities, not because of their actions but because of their wealth, he noted. Moreover, he said, even if the progression of climate change leads to lost food sources and creates climate migrants, the wealthiest people will likely continue to have adequate resources. He asked about efforts to address equity issues and to change the behavior of the richest 1 percent, who control vast amounts of wealth in the United States and around the world. Barrangou replied that some extremely wealthy people have funded organizations to address broad issues, such as the Jeff Bezos Earth Fund, the Bill and Melinda Gates Foundation, and the Chan Zuckerberg Initiative. He characterized these as exemplary models of using influence and wealth to drive data-informed decisions, influence policies, and channel resources to solving substantial problems. These organizations foster social and science solutions that adopt a global perspective to help a large number of people, said Barrangou. Malshe commented that in the last 20–30 years, digital technologies have lifted many people out of poverty, with affluence reflected in worldwide obesity. He suggested that policies focusing on the middle 60 percent of the socioeconomic sector of society could yield real change for nutritional food habits.

CLOSING REMARKS

Barrangou thanked all Food Forum members, past and present, and symposium participants and contributors. He underscored the highly complex problems related to the food system that affect large numbers of key players. Both concern and optimism are present in the forum, he said, which comprises the "right people, the right place, and the right time" to address the myriad issues highlighted at the symposium. Satisfaction with the accomplishments of the forum over the past three decades can offer momentum for continued problem-solving of the grand challenges faced today, Barrangou concluded.

References

Adams, S. H., J. C. Anthony, R. Carvajal, L. Chae, C. San, H. Khoo, M. E. Latulippe, N. V. Matusheski, H. L. McClung, M. Rozga, C. H. Schmid, S. Wopereis, and W. Yan. 2020. Perspective: Guiding principles for the implementation of personalized nutrition approaches that benefit health and function. *Advances in Nutrition* 11(1):25-34. https://doi.org/10.1093/advances/nmz086.

Agricultural Research Service. 2019. *FoodData Central.* U.S. Department of Agriculture. https://fdc.nal.usda.gov/ (accessed February 23, 2024).

ATSDR (Agency for Toxic Substances and Disease Registry). 2024. 2024. *PFAS (per- and polyfluoroalkyl substances) in people in the United States over time.* Centers for Disease Control and Prevention. https://www.atsdr.cdc.gov/pfas/health-effects/us-population.html (accessed February 23, 2024).

Atwater, W. O., and D. Chas. 1896. *The chemical composition of American food materials.* https://www.ars.usda.gov/ARSUserFiles/80400530/pdf/hist/oes_1896_bul_28.pdf (accessed February 23, 2024).

Béné, C., P. Oosterveer, L. Lamotte, I. D. Brouwer, S. Haan, S. D. Prager, E. F. Talsma, and C. K. Khoury. 2019. When food systems meet sustainability—Current narratives and implications for actions. *World Development* 113:116-130.

Brown, A. F., G. X. Ma, J. Miranda, E. Eng, D. Castille, T. Brockie, P. Jones, C. O. Airhihenbuwa, T. Farhat, L. Zhu, and C. Trinh-Shevrin. 2019. Structural interventions to reduce and eliminate health disparities. *American Journal of Public Health* 109(S1):S72-S78.

Buttorff, C., T. Ruder, and M. Bauma. 2023. *Health and economic costs of chronic diseases.* Centers for Disease Control and Prevention. https://www.cdc.gov/chronicdisease/about/costs/index.htm (accessed February 23, 2024).

Crippa, M., E. Solazzo, D. Guizzardi, F. Monforti-Ferrario, F. N. Tubiello, and A. Leip. 2021. Food systems are responsible for a third of global anthropogenic GHG (greenhouse gas) emissions. *Nature Food* 2:198-209. https://doi.org/10.1038/s43016-021-00225-9.

Didion, J. 1968. *Slouching towards Bethlehem: Essays.* New York: Farrar, Straus and Giroux.

Fanzo, J., A. L. Bellows, M. L. Spiker, A. L. Thorne-Lyman, and M. W. Bloem. 2021. The importance of food systems and the environment for nutrition. *American Journal of Clinical Nutrition* 113(1):7-16.

FDA (Food and Drug Administration). n.d. *Survey data on acrylamide in food.* www.fda.gov/food/process-contaminants-food/survey-data-acrylamide-food (accessed April 30, 2024).

FDA. 2023. *Whole genome sequencing (WGS) program.* https://www.fda.gov/food/microbiology-research-food/whole-genome-sequencing-wgs-program (accessed February 23, 2024).

Goldenberg, S. M., R. M. Thomas, A. Forbes, and S. Baral. 2021. *Sex work, health, and human rights: Global inequities, challenges, and opportunities for action.* Cham: Springer.

He, J., Z. Zhu, J. D. Bundy, K. S. Dorans, J. Chen, and L. L. Hamm. 2015. Trends in cardiovascular risk factors in U.S. adults by race and ethnicity and socioeconomic status. *Journal of the American Medical Association* 326(13):1286-1298. https://doi.org/10.1001/jama.2021.15187.

Japsen, B. 2020, December 8. Poor worker health costs U.S. employers $575 billion a year. *Forbes.* https://www.forbes.com/sites/brucejapsen/2020/12/08/poor-worker-health-costs-us-employers-575-billion-a-year/?sh=baaa64217b2f (accessed February 23, 2024).

Li, J., A. Scarano, N. M. Gonzalez, F. D'Orso, Y. Yue, K. Nemeth, G. Saalbach, L. Hill, C. O. Martins, R. Moran, A. Santino, and C. Martin. 2022. Biofortified tomatoes provide a new route to vitamin D sufficiency. *Nature Plants* 8:611-616. https://doi.org/10.1038/s41477-022-01154-6.

Meadows, D. H. 2008. *Thinking in systems—A primer.* White River Junction, VT: Chelsea Green Publishing.

NHGRI (National Human Genome Research Institute). 2023. *The Human Genome Project.* National Institutes of Health, U.S. Department of Health and Human Services, Office of Science, and U.S Department of Energy. https://www.genome.gov/human-genome-project (accessed February 23, 2024).

Ordovas, J. M., L. R. Ferguson, E. S. Tai, and J. C. Mathers. 2018. Personalised nutrition and health. *British Medical Journal* 361. https://doi.org/10.1136/bmj.k2173.

Parsons, K., C. Hawkes, and R. Wells. 2019. *What is the food system? A food policy perspective.* Centre for Food Policy, City University of London. https://www.city.ac.uk/__data/assets/pdf_file/0004/570442/7643_Brief-2_What-is-the-food-system-A-food-policy-perspective_WEB_SP.pdf (accessed February 23, 2024).

Rich, N. 2018, August 1. Losing Earth: The decade we almost stopped climate change. *The New York Times Magazine.* https://www.nytimes.com/interactive/2018/08/01/magazine/climate-change-losing-earth.html (accessed May 14, 2024).

Ritchie, H., and M. Roser. 2019. Land use. *Our World in Data.* https://ourworldindata.org/land-use (accessed February 23, 2024).

Ritchie, H., P. Rosado, and M. Roser. 2022. What are the environmental impacts of food and agriculture? *Our World in Data.* https://ourworldindata.org/environmental-impacts-of-food (accessed February 23, 2024).

Solar, O., and A. Irwin. 2010. *A conceptual framework for action on the social determinants of health.* Social Determinants of Health Discussion Paper. World Health Organization. https://www.who.int/publications/i/item/9789241500852 (accessed February 23, 2024).

Steffen, W., K. Richardson, J. Rockstrom, S. E. Cornell, I. Fetzer, E. M. Bennett, R. Biggs, S. R. Carpenter, W. Vries, C. A. Wit, C. Folke, D. Gerten, J. Heike, G. M. Mace, L. M. Persson, V. Ramanathan, B. Reyes, and S. Sorlin. 2015. Planetary boundaries: Guiding human development on a changing planet. *Science* 347(6223). http://dx.doi.org/10.1126/science.1259855.

Tillotson, J. E. 2004. America's obesity: Conflicting public policies, industrial economic development, and unintended human consequences. *Annual Review of Nutrition* 24(1):617-643. https://scholar.archive.org/work/amcympkuengvdhzffkcrzafgla/access/wayback/http:/www.farmpolicy.com:80/annurev.nutr24012003132434.pdf (accessed February 23, 2024).

UKRI (UK Research Institute). 2023, August 7. *UKRI food deep dive summary report.* UKRI Food Safety Research Network. fsrn.quadram.ac.uk/app/uploads/2023/09/9924_UKRI-Food-Deep-Dive-Summary-Report_v2_CB_compressed.pdf (accessed April 30, 2024).

Watson, K. B., S. A. Carlson, F. Loustalot, J. E. Fulton, D. Galuska, J. M. Dorn, and J. E. Fulton. 2022. Chronic conditions among adults aged 18–34 years—Behavioral Risk Factor Surveillance System, United States, 2019. *Morbidity and Mortality Weekly Report* 71(30): 964-970.

Wilkinson, M., M. Dumontier, and I. Aalbersberg. 2016. The FAIR Guiding Principles for scientific data management and stewardship. *Scientific Data* 3, 160018. https://doi.org/10.1038/sdata.2016.18.

Wood, A., C. Queiroz, L. Deutsch, B. González-Mon, M. Jonell, L. Pereira, H. Sinare, U. Svedin, and E. Wassénius. 2023. Reframing the local–global food systems debate through a resilience lens. *Nature Food* 4(1):22-29. https://doi.org/10.1038/s43016-022-00662-0.

World Obesity Federation. 2023. *World obesity atlas 2023.* https://data.worldobesity.org/publications/WOF-Obesity-Atlas-V5.pdf (accessed February 23, 2024).

Appendix A

Symposium Agenda

Food Forum 30th Anniversary Symposium
November 30, 2023

SETTING THE STAGE:
THE FOOD FORUM'S INFLUENCE AND IMPACT

9:00 AM ET   **Opening Remarks**
Monica N. Feit, Ph.D., M.P.H., *Executive Director*,
Health and Medicine Division, National Academies of
Sciences, Engineering, and Medicine
Marcia McNutt, Ph.D., *President*, National Academy of
Sciences
Eric A. Decker, Ph.D., M.S., *Food Forum Chair*,
Professor, Department of Food Science, University of
Massachusetts Amherst

9:20 AM ET   **History of the Food Forum and Its Impact Over the Past**
30 Years
Eric A. Decker, Ph.D., M.S., Professor, Department of
Food Science, University of Massachusetts Amherst,
Food Forum Chair since 2022
Sylvia Rowe, M.A.T., President, SR Strategy, *Food*
Forum Chair 2015–2021

Francis (Frank) F. Busta, Ph.D., M.S., Director Emeritus, National Center for Food Protection and Defense (now Food Protection & Defense Institute), Professor Emeritus, University of Minnesota, *Food Forum Chair 2011–2014*

Michael P. Doyle, Ph.D., M.S., Retired Regents Professor, Director, Center for Food Safety, University of Georgia, *Food Forum Chair 2003–2011*

Fergus (Ferg) M. Clydesdale, Ph.D., M.A., Distinguished University Professor, Department of Food Science, University of Massachusetts Amherst, *Food Forum Chair 1996–2002*

9:40 AM ET   **Break**

THIRTY YEARS OF THE FOOD FORUM: REFLECTING ON PROGRESS, ENVISIONING THE ROAD AHEAD

10:00 AM ET   **Key Area: Food Safety**
Moderator: Sam R. Nugen, Ph.D., Professor, Department of Food Science, Cornell University

Susan T. Mayne, Ph.D., Former Director, Center for Food Safety and Applied Nutrition, U.S. Food and Drug Administration

Stefanie N. Evans, Ph.D., Vice President, Food Safety, Quality, and Regulatory Affairs, Conagra Brands, Inc.

Haley Oliver, Ph.D., 150th Anniversary Professor, Assistant Dean for Online Programs, College of Agriculture, Director, U.S. Agency for International Development Feed the Future Food Safety Innovation Lab, Purdue University

30-minute Panel Discussion

11:00 AM ET   **Key Area: Food Systems and Sustainability**
Moderator: Christina Khoo, Ph.D., Director, Emerging Science, Nutrition, and Regulatory Affairs, Ocean Spray Cranberries, Inc.

Jessica Fanzo, Ph.D., M.S., Professor, Director, Food for Humanity Initiative, Climate School, Columbia University

Stephanie K. Goodwin, Ph.D., M.P.H., R.D., Director, Nutrition Policy, Danone North America

Christian Peters, Ph.D., M.S., Research Leader, Food Systems Research Unit, Agricultural Research Service, U.S. Department of Agriculture
30-minute Panel Discussion

12:00 PM ET   Lunch

1:15 PM ET   **Key Area: Nutrition & Health**
Moderator: Christina Khoo, Ph.D., Director, Emerging Science, Nutrition, and Regulatory Affairs, Ocean Spray Cranberries, Inc.
Josh Anthony, Ph.D., M.B.A., M.S., Founder and CEO, Nlumn
Naomi K. Fukagawa, M.D., Ph.D., Director, Beltsville Human Nutrition Research Center, Agricultural Research Service, U.S. Department of Agriculture, Professor of Medicine Emerita, University of Vermont
Angela Odoms-Young, Ph.D., M.S., The Nancy Schlegel Meinig Associate Professor of Maternal and Child Nutrition, Director, Food and Nutrition Education in Communities Program and New York State Expanded Food and Nutrition Education Program, Cornell University
30-minute Panel Discussion

2:15 PM ET   **Break**

2:30 PM ET   **A Visionary Perspective on the Future of Food**
Guy Poppy, D.Phil, CB, FMedSci, Executive Chair, Biotechnology and Biological Sciences Research Council, Executive Sponsor of Food Research and Innovation, UK Research and Innovation

3:00 PM ET   **Fireside Chat: Food for Thought on the Next 30 Years**
Moderator: Rodolphe Barrangou, Ph.D., M.B.A., M.S., Todd R. Klaenhammer Distinguished Professor in Probiotics Research, Department of Food Bioprocessing and Nutrition Sciences, North Carolina State University
Panelists:
• Lauren Abda, M.S., Founder and CEO, Branchfood, Cofounder, Branch Venture Group

- Ajay P. Malshe, Ph.D., R. Eugene and Susie E. Goodson Distinguished Professor of Mechanical Engineering, and Agricultural and Biological Engineering, Purdue University
- Susan T. Mayne, Ph.D., Former Director, Center for Food Safety and Applied Nutrition, U.S. Food and Drug Administration
- Xavier Morales, Ph.D., M.R.P., Executive Director, The Praxis Project
- Guy Poppy, D.Phil, C.B., FmedSci, Executive Chair, Biotechnology and Biological Sciences Research Council, Executive Sponsor of Food Research and Innovation, UK Research and Innovation

4:00 PM ET   **Adjourn**

Appendix B

Biographical Sketches of Symposium Speakers and Planning Committee Members

Lauren Abda, M.S., is founder and CEO of Branchfood, a launchpad for food innovation and one of the largest communities of food innovators in the world. She is also cofounder of Branch Venture Group, one of the first angel investment networks focused exclusively on funding agri-foodtech startups in the United States. Ms. Abda is a council member at the Tufts University Nutrition Innovation Institute; she is on the board of advisors for the Boston Public Market Association; and she has served as a mentor and judge for leading startup programs, including the Rabobank–MIT Food & Agribusiness Innovation Prize and MassChallenge. Prior to her entrepreneurial endeavors, she consulted for agri-foodtech businesses in Boston and San Francisco; worked as an analyst for Salt Venture Partners, a corporate venture capital firm within the Harvard Common Press; and wrote reports on international food safety development initiatives on behalf of the Agriculture and Commodities division at the World Trade Organization in Geneva, Switzerland. Ms. Abda has a B.S. in nutrition and food science from the University of Vermont and an M.S. in food policy and applied nutrition from the Tufts Friedman School of Nutrition Science and Policy.

Josh Anthony, Ph.D., M.B.A., M.S., is founder and CEO of Nlumn, a business-to-business personalized nutrition and health consulting company. Before starting Nlumn, Dr. Anthony was founding chief science officer at the personalized nutrition company Habit. He was also vice president of global nutrition and health at the Campbell Soup Company. Prior to Habit and Campbell, he held progressive technical and management roles at Reckitt-Mead Johnson Nutrition and Unilever. He also served as an adjunct professor of physiology at the Indiana University School of Medicine. Over the past 25 years working in the food and nutrition business with Fortune 500 companies and startups, Dr. Anthony has proven his capabilities as a successful scientist, innovator, and entrepreneur. Driven by the challenge of translating science to help people achieve their health and wellness goals, he has worked collaboratively to help launch more than 150 science-based products and services supported by more than 140 patents. He is a trusted board member and advisor to executives across food, nutrition, and ingredient companies, universities, and not-for-profit organizations. Dr. Anthony earned a B.S. in biological sciences from Carnegie Mellon University, an M.S. in nutritional sciences from the University of Illinois, a Ph.D. in cell and molecular physiology from the Pennsylvania State University College of Medicine, and an M.B.A. from Vanderbilt University.

Douglas Balentine, Ph.D., is senior science advisor for international nutrition policy at the Food and Drug Administration's (FDA's) Center for Food Safety and Applied Nutrition (CFSAN) (2019–current). In this role, he supports the critical work of the Codex Alimentarius as the U.S. delegate to both the Codex Committee on Nutrition and Foods for Special Dietary Use and the Codex Committee on Food Labeling. In addition, Dr. Balentine leads international activities and multilateral issues related to FDA's nutrition and food labeling programs. This includes authoritative scientific and policy advice and guidance, and recommendations on international nutrition activities and programs, considering input from U.S. stakeholders while advancing FDA's science-based public health mission. Formerly, Dr. Balentine served as director of the Office of Nutrition and Food Labeling at CFSAN from 2015 to 2019; in that role, he provided leadership and scientific direction to a multidisciplinary staff that managed regulatory programs relating to food labeling, nutrition, infant formula, and medical foods. Prior to joining FDA, he served as director of Nutrition and Health for Unilever North America and was a member of Unilever's Global Nutrition Leadership Team. Dr. Balentine has worked closely with many organizations and served on a number of committees with goals of improving public health. He holds 15 patents and has more than 40 publications in scientific literature. Dr. Balentine has a Ph.D. in food science and nutrition from Rutgers University.

Rodolphe Barrangou, Ph.D., M.B.A., M.S., is T. R. Klaenhammer distinguished professor in probiotics research in the Department of Food, Bioprocessing and Nutrition Sciences at North Carolina State University, focusing on the evolution and functions of CRISPR-Cas systems and their applications in bacteria used in food manufacturing. He spent 9 years in research and development and mergers and acquisitions at Danisco and

DuPont in the food industry. Recently, for his work establishing the biological function of CRISPR, Dr. Barrangou received the 2016 Warren Alpert Prize, the 2016 Canada Gairdner International Award, the 2017 National Academy of Sciences (NAS) Award in Molecular Biology, and the 2018 NAS Prize in Food and Agriculture Sciences. He was elected to the NAS in 2018 and the National Academy of Engineering in 2019, as well as the National Academy of Inventors and the National Inventors Hall of Fame. Dr. Barrangou is also former chairman of the board of directors of Caribou Biosciences; cofounder of Intellia Therapeutics, Locus Biosciences, CRISPR Biotechnologies, Ancilia Biosciences, and TreeCo; and editor-in-chief of CRISPR Journal. He holds a B.S. in biological sciences from René Descartes University in Paris, France; an M.B.A. from the University of Wisconsin–Madison; an M.S. in biological engineering from the University of Technology in Compiègne, France; and an M.S. in food science and Ph.D. in genomics from North Carolina State University.

Francis (Frank) F. Busta, Ph.D., M.S., is director emeritus of the National Center for Food Protection and Defense (NCFPD; now Food Protection & Defense Institute) and professor emeritus of food microbiology at the University of Minnesota. Dr. Busta's research areas are in food safety, growth and survival of microorganisms after environmental stress in food, microbial ecology, and food defense. He published more than 125 refereed research papers. Previously, Dr. Busta held faculty positions at the University of Minnesota, North Carolina State University, and the University of Florida. He served as chair of the Department of Food Science and Human Nutrition from 1984 to 1987 at the University of Florida and head of the Department of Food Science & Nutrition at the University of Minnesota from 1987 to 1997. He became professor emeritus in 1999. Dr. Busta retired in 2002 from the International Commission on the Microbiological Specifications for Food after 15 years of service. He is a fellow of the Institute of Food Technologists (IFT) and was president from 1995 to 1996. He is also a fellow of the American Academy of Microbiology, the American Association for the Advancement of Science, the Institute of Food Science and Technology (IFST in the United Kingdom), the International Association for Food Protection (IAFP), and the Academy of the International Union of Food Science and Technology, and he has received additional awards from several of these organizations. He chaired the Food Forum of the National Academies of Sciences, Engineering, and Medicine from 2011 to 2014. He is a certified food scientist and a registered scientist. Dr. Busta received his B.A. and M.S. from the University of Minnesota and his Ph.D. from the University of Illinois.

Fergus (Ferg) M. Clydesdale, Ph.D., M.A., is distinguished university professor in the Department of Food Science at the University of Massachusetts

Amherst and was director of the University of Massachusetts Food Science Policy Alliance from 2005 to 2020. From 1988 to 2008, he was head of the Department of Food Science. His research involves the role of technology in creating healthy and sustainable diets and its regulation and policy. Dr. Clydesdale is a fellow of five premier societies in the field of food science and nutrition, is editor-in-chief of *Critical Reviews in Food Science and Nutrition*, and has published some 375 scientific articles and coauthored or edited 20 books. He has held professorships and has given invited presentations around the globe and has been an invited speaker in the National Academy of Sciences Distinctive Voices Series at the Jonsson Center. Dr. Clydesdale also has served on or chaired numerous committees of the Institute of Food Technologists (IFT), the U.S. Food and Drug Administration, the International Life Sciences Institute (ILSI), and the International Food Information Council (IFIC). At the National Academies of Sciences, Engineering, and Medicine, he served on the Food and Nutrition Board and chaired the Food Forum from 1996 to 2002. He also served on the 2005 Dietary Guidelines Advisory Committee and on the board of trustees of ILSI and IFIC. He is the recipient of innumerable awards, including IFT's highest honor, the Nicolas Appert Award. The University of Massachusetts Amherst has established the Fergus M. Clydesdale professorship and dedicated the Fergus M. Clydesdale Center for Foods for Health and Wellness in 2011 in his honor. Dr. Clydesdale received his M.A. in food chemistry from the University of Toronto and his Ph.D. in food science and technology from the University of Massachusetts Amherst.

Eric A. Decker, Ph.D., M.S., (Chair), is professor of food science at the University of Massachusetts Amherst. He has also been director of the UMass Food Science Industry Strategic Research Alliance since 2008. Dr. Decker is actively conducting research to characterize mechanisms of lipid oxidation, antioxidant protection of foods, and the health implications of bioactive lipids. He has more than 430 publications and has been listed as one of the Most Highly Cited Scientists in Agriculture since 2005. Dr. Decker has served on numerous committees for institutions such as the Food and Drug Administration; National Academies of Sciences, Engineering, and Medicine; Institute of Food Technologists; U.S. Department of Agriculture; and American Heart Association. He has received recognition for his research and service from the American Oil Chemist Society, Agriculture and Food Chemistry Division of the American Chemical Society, Institute of Food Technologists, University of Massachusetts, and University of Kentucky. Dr. Decker has also been elected to serve as an officer for the American Meat Science Association and Institute of Food Technologists, and, most recently, as president of the American Oil Chemist Society. He holds an M.S. in food science and nutrition from Washington State

University and a Ph.D. in food science and nutrition from the University of Massachusetts Amherst.

Michael P. Doyle, Ph.D., M.S., is retired regent's professor and director of the Center for Food Safety at the University of Georgia Griffin. From 1977 to 1980, he was senior project leader of corporate microbiology at Ralston Purina Company, and from 1980 to 1991 he advanced from assistant professor to Wisconsin distinguished professor of food microbiology at the Food Research Institute at the University of Wisconsin–Madison. Dr. Doyle has been a leading researcher in microbiological food safety and worked closely with the food industry, government agencies, and consumer groups on issues related to the microbiological safety of foods. He published more than 500 scientific papers on food microbiology and food safety topics, and has given more than 900 invited presentations at national and international scientific meetings. He has served on food safety committees of many scientific organizations and has been a scientific advisor to many groups, including the World Health Organization, International Life Sciences Institute, U.S. Food and Drug Administration, U.S. Department of Agriculture, U.S. Department of Defense, U.S. Environmental Protection Agency, and many leading national and international food companies. Dr. Doyle is a member of the National Academy of Medicine, has served as a member and chair of numerous committees at the National Academies, and was chair of the Food Forum from 2003 to 2011. He has received many awards for his research accomplishments, including the Nicholas Appert Award of the Institute of Food Technologists (IFT). He is a fellow of the American Academy of Microbiology, the American Association for the Advancement of Science, IFT, the International Association for Food Protection, and the National Academy of Inventors. Dr. Doyle received his B.S., M.S., and Ph.D. degrees from the University of Wisconsin–Madison in bacteriology/food microbiology.

Stefanie N. Evans, Ph.D., is vice president of food safety, quality, and regulatory affairs at Conagra Brands, Inc. In this role, she leads an experienced and talented team of microbiologists, chemists, and quality, sanitation, regulatory, and thermal process specialists who support Conagra's manufacturing facilities, comanufacturers, and suppliers. Dr. Evans has 20 years of experience and consulting in the food industry across large companies and small startups in broad categories of food and beverages, including ready-to-eat, frozen, plant-based, fermented, and organic products. She previously spent 5 years with Conagra Brands and rejoined in 2021 after 7 years in positions with WhiteWave Foods, Danone North America, Kite Hill, and small startups. She has developed expertise in food manufacturing, quality systems, risk management, and delivering quality products to the market. Dr. Evans has a Ph.D. in food safety microbiology from the University of Nebraska.

Jessica Fanzo, Ph.D., M.S., is professor of climate and director of the Food for Humanity Initiative at Columbia University's Climate School in New York City. She also serves as interim director for the International Research Institute for Climate and Society. She has held positions at Johns Hopkins University, the Food and Agriculture Organization (FAO) of the United Nations (UN), the UN World Food Programme, Bioversity International, the Earth Institute, the Millennium Development Goal Centre at the World Agroforestry Center in Kenya, and the Doris Duke Charitable Foundation. She has participated in various collective endeavors, including the Food Systems Economic Commission, the Global Panel of Agriculture and Food Systems for Nutrition Foresight 2.0 report, the Lancet Commission on Anaemia, and the EAT-Lancet Commissions 1 and 2. She was also co-chair of the Global Nutrition Report and team leader for the UN High-Level Panel of Experts on Food Systems and Nutrition. Dr. Fanzo currently leads the development of the Food Systems Dashboard and the Food Systems Countdown to 2030 Initiative in collaboration with the Global Alliance of Improved Nutrition and FAO. She holds an M.S. and Ph.D. from the University of Arizona.

Monica N. Feit, Ph.D., M.P.H., is executive director of the Health and Medicine Division at the National Academies of Sciences, Engineering, and Medicine. She has been with the National Academies in various roles for almost 15 years, including as a senior program officer who staffed reports on LGBT health and integrating primary care and public health. She led an initiative on innovation and launched the Societal Experts Action Network, which brought together social science experts to respond to urgent questions related to COVID-19. In addition, Dr. Feit was a member of the Senior Executive Service in the U.S. Department of Health and Human Services, where she held leadership positions at the Substance Abuse and Mental Health Services Administration and the Office of the Assistant Secretary for Planning and Evaluation. She served as an American Public Health Association fellow on the Senate Committee on Health, Education, Labor, and Pensions and worked in international health for many years, including in Bosnia and Herzegovina, Niger, and South Africa. She received her B.A. from Smith College, M.P.H. from Columbia University, and Ph.D. from London South Bank University.

Naomi K. Fukagawa, M.D., Ph.D., is director of the U.S. Department of Agriculture (USDA) Agricultural Research Service's (ARS) Beltsville Human Nutrition Research Center and professor of medicine emerita at the University of Vermont (UVM). She is a board-certified pediatrician with expertise in nutritional biochemistry and metabolism, including protein and energy metabolism, oxidants and antioxidants, and the role of diet in aging and chronic diseases. She was president of the American Society for Clinical Nutrition and the American Society for Nutrition and served as vice chair of the 2010 Dietary Guidelines Advisory Committee. She served as associate editor of the *American Journal of Clinical Nutrition* and editor-in-chief of *Nutrition Reviews*. Her clinical training included residency at the Children's Hospital of Philadelphia at the University of Pennsylvania, chief residency at UVM, and nutrition/gerontology fellowships at the Children's Hospital and Beth Israel Hospital at the Harvard Medical School (HMS). She was assistant professor at HMS and the Massachusetts Institute of Technology (MIT), serving as director of the Nutrition Support Service at the Boston Children's Hospital. She was also assistant professor at the Rockefeller University and served as the associate director of the Clinical Research Centers at MIT, Rockefeller University, and UVM. She continues research ranging from cells and animals to in vivo studies in human volunteers with a focus on the impact of environmental stressors (metabolic or physical) on health, specifically the impact of exposure to particulate matter generated from the combustion of petrodiesel and biodiesel fuels. As a leader of the team responsible for the USDA ARS FoodData Central, an integrated food composition data system, she promotes environmentally friendly and sustainable food production and supports accessible, affordable, and nutritious food supply for all. She received her Ph.D. from MIT and M.D. from Northwestern University.

Stephanie K. Goodwin, Ph.D., M.P.H., R.D., is director of nutrition policy for the public affairs and government team at Danone North America. Danone is a purpose-driven global food and beverage manufacturer and in North America is a public benefit corporation, and a proud Certified B Corporation® with the mission of "health through food to as many people as possible." She has been with Danone for 9 years, first on the science team, and then on the regulatory affairs team. Prior to joining Danone, Dr. Goodwin worked within the Office of the Assistant Secretary for Health, U.S. Department of Health and Human Services, on the 2015 Dietary Guidelines supporting the Advisory Committee on Sustainable Diets. She is a registered dietitian, and she earned an M.P.H. in health education and a Ph.D. in human nutrition and public policy from the Virginia Polytechnic Institute and State University. She completed her postdoctoral fellowship in metabolic science at the National Institutes of Health.

Christina Khoo, Ph.D., is director of emerging science, nutrition, and regulatory affairs at Ocean Spray Cranberries, Inc. She leads a team responsible for providing scientific substantiation for the development of functional health products and regulatory guidance for messaging and claims. During her tenure, Dr. Khoo successfully obtained the first Food and Drug Administration–qualified health claim for a food (cranberry) to help reduce an acute urinary tract infection. She also led initiatives on novel foods and Generally Recognized As Safe approvals. Dr. Khoo is also responsible for emerging science and technology scouting, spearheading several projects with startup companies, and evaluating technologies "from farm to fork" to help accelerate innovation and sustainability initiatives. As an influencer, she has taken on leadership roles in cross-sector initiatives, such as chair of the Institute for the Advancement of Food and Nutrition Sciences bioactives committee and the cognitive health working group. She also serves as treasurer of the National Berry Crops Alliance board and is currently chair of the Juice Products Association Board of Directors. Dr. Khoo participates actively as a member of the National Academies of Sciences, Engineering, and Medicine's Food Forum, as well as the Tufts Friedman School's Food and Nutrition Innovation Institute as the co-chair of the bioactives working group, where she collaborates with cross-sector partners to work on important food and nutrition issues. Dr. Khoo received her doctorate from the Food Science and Human Nutrition Department at the University of Florida and completed a postdoctoral fellowship at Harvard T. H. Chan School of Public Health's Department of Nutrition.

Ajay P. Malshe, Ph.D., is R. Eugene and Susie E. Goodson distinguished professor of mechanical engineering and agriculture and biological engineering (by courtesy) at Purdue University. He is inaugural director of the Materials and Manufacturing Research Laboratories and codirector of Purdue's Engineering Initiative for eXcellence in Manufacturing and Operations. Areas of his core competencies are advanced manufacturing, multifunctional-resilient-sustainable bioinspired designing, functional multimaterials, frugal engineering, and system integration and productization. Over the decades, application areas of his interest and contributions are biomanufacturing for future foods and farms at the point of need, heterogeneous microelectronics for high-density systems, nanomanufacturing for extreme machines, in-space servicing, assembly, and manufacturing. Dr. Malshe has trained more than 1,400 graduate and undergraduate students, published more than 225 peer-reviewed manuscripts, and received more than 28 patents. His patents resulted in more than 20 award-winning engineered products applied by leading corporations around the world. Dr. Malshe serves multiple professional organizations in various roles as a committee member and board member. For example, he is a member of Sci-Tech Advisory Board of Good Food Institute and a committee member in the Responsive Agriculture Study, Texas A&M University Institute for Advancing Health Through

Agriculture, and the Chicago Council on Global Affairs. He is a member of the National Academy of Engineering, and he has received more than 45 international honors for scientific discoveries, engineering innovations, and breakthrough products. Dr. Malshe holds a Ph.D. in physics from Savitribai Phule Pune University in Maharashtra, India, and completed his post doctorate at The Ohio State University.

Susan T. Mayne, Ph.D., is former director of the Center for Food Safety and Applied Nutrition (CFSAN) at the U.S. Food and Drug Administration (FDA). Serving in this position from January 2015 to May 2023, Dr. Mayne led the Center's development and implementation of programs and policies related to the safety and labeling of foods covering approximately 80 percent of the U.S. food supply. During her tenure as CFSAN director, the Center advanced landmark food safety and nutrition policies including the implementation of the FDA Food Safety Modernization Act (FSMA), Closer to Zero to reduce toxic elements in foods for babies and young children, trans fat reduction, updating the iconic nutrition facts label to include added sugars, issuing sodium reduction targets for industry across more than 160 categories of food, and implementing menu labeling so consumers can access calorie and nutrition information when consuming foods away from home. Prior to joining the FDA, she spent nearly three decades at Yale University, where she held an endowed chair as the C.-E.A. Winslow professor of epidemiology and served as chair of the Department of Chronic Disease Epidemiology and associate director of the Yale Cancer Center. Dr. Mayne is author/coauthor of nearly 250 scientific publications, and her work has been cited more than 17,000 times. She completed two terms on the Food and Nutrition Board of the National Academy of Sciences and served on numerous committees, including committees to establish Dietary Reference Intakes, prior to joining the FDA. Dr. Mayne received a B.A. in chemistry from the University of Colorado and a Ph.D. in nutritional sciences, with minors in biochemistry and toxicology, from Cornell University.

Marcia McNutt, Ph.D., is a geophysicist and the 22nd president of the National Academy of Sciences. From 2013 to 2016, she was editor-in-chief of Science journals. Dr. McNutt was director of the U.S. Geological Survey (USGS) from 2009 to 2013, during which time USGS responded to a number of major disasters, including the Deepwater Horizon oil spill. For her work to help contain that spill, she was awarded the U.S. Coast Guard's Meritorious Service Medal. Dr. McNutt is a fellow of the American Geophysical Union (AGU), Geological Society of America, the American Association for the Advancement of Science, and the International Association of Geodesy. She is a member of the National Academy of Engineering, the American Philosophical Society, and the American Academy of Arts and Sciences; a foreign member of the U.K. Royal Society, the Russian Academy of Sciences, and the Chinese Academy of Sciences; and a foreign fellow of the Indian National Science Academy. In 1998, Dr. McNutt was awarded the AGU's Macelwane Medal for research accomplishments by a young scientist, and she received the Maurice Ewing Medal in 2007 for her contributions to deep-sea exploration. She holds a B.A. in physics from Colorado College and Ph.D. in earth sciences from the Scripps Institution of Oceanography.

Xavier Morales, Ph.D., M.R.P., is executive director for the Praxis Project, a national organization that centers equity and community power in efforts to transform policies, systems, structures, and practices that underlie inequity and injustice. Before Praxis, he led the Latino Coalition for a Healthy California. At both organizations, Dr. Morales has worked to center health, equity, and racial justice as a foundation for organizational goals and strategies. While adopting and advocating for a Learning Circle/Community of Practice approach to accompany power-building partners in their efforts to address community-defined justice priorities, he strives for the Praxis Project's work to be less extractive and to create a space for bidirectional learning where all expertise is heard and valued. Dr. Morales has spent the last 20 years learning from community advocates; before that, he received a B.A. in environmental science from the University of California, Berkeley, and an M.R.P. and Ph.D. from Cornell University's Department of City and Regional Planning.

Megan Nechanicky, M.S., R.D., joined General Mills in 2014 and is currently nutrition manager for North America Retail and Global Health & Wellness communications. In her role, her team provides strategic direction for business and research and development partners related to health and wellness. She also leads a team focused on communications with stakeholders on the company's nutrition commitments and advancements, and works externally with government, trade associations, and academic institutions to positively position General Mills for future growth. In 2017, Ms. Nechanicky completed a 6-month international assignment in the General Mills Nyon, Switzerland, office where she gained experience living and working within the Europe and Australian Region to build and advance nutrition science, research, and communications. When she first joined General Mills, Ms. Nechanicky led health influencer communications for some of General Mills's largest brands, including Cheerios®, Fiber One®, and Nature Valley®. In this role, she delivered cutting-edge science, consumer trends, and new product development and marketing to health influencers such as dietitians, physicians, nurses, and fitness professionals. Prior to General Mills, she was the first dietitian to work at the President's Council on Sports, Fitness & Nutrition. In her role, Ms. Nechanicky led nutrition and physical activity–related initiatives and events. She was also responsible for the Department of Health and Human Services coordination of First Lady Michelle Obama's Let's Move! initiative to end childhood obesity within a generation. She also served on the federal steering committee to develop the U.S. Department of Health and Human Services Physical Activity Guidelines Midcourse Report and coordinated the communications strategy and report launch in 2013. Ms. Nechanicky is a registered dietitian and holds a bachelor's degree in food marketing from Saint Joseph's University in Philadelphia, Pennsylvania, and a dual master's degree in exercise physiology and nutrition from San Diego State University.

Sam R. Nugen, Ph.D., is professor of food and biosystems engineering in the Department of Food Science at Cornell University and was previously assistant professor at the University of Massachusetts Amherst. His research group utilizes synthetic biology and phage-based biosensors to develop novel methods for separating and detecting pathogens from complex matrices such as food and environmental samples. Previously, he was research engineer at Kraft Foods. Dr. Nugen received his B.S. in animal science from the University of Vermont and M.S. and Ph.D. in food science from Cornell University. He completed his postdoctoral work in the Department of Biological Engineering at Cornell.

Angela Odoms-Young, Ph.D., M.S., is Nancy Schlegel Meinig associate professor of maternal and child nutrition at Cornell University, and director of the Food and Nutrition Education in Communities program and New York State Expanded Food and Nutrition Education Program. Prior to joining Cornell, Dr. Odoms-Young served on the faculty at the University of Illinois Chicago in the Department of Kinesiology and Nutrition. Her research explores social and structural determinants of dietary behaviors and diet-related diseases in low-income and Black/Latinx populations and centers on identifying culturally appropriate programs and policies that promote health equity, food justice, and community resilience. Dr. Odoms-Young has more than 20 years of experience partnering with communities to improve nutrition and health and more than 200 academic publications, book chapters, and presentations. She has served on numerous advisory committees and boards, including the National Academies of Sciences, Engineering, and Medicine Food and Nutrition Board; Institute of Medicine (now Health and Medicine Division) committees to develop the nutrition standards for the National School Lunch Program/School Breakfast Program and revise the food packages provided in the Supplemental Program for Women, Infants, and Children; and Council on Black Health. Dr. Odoms-Young has also been a member of the board of the Greater Chicago Food Depository (previous), American Heart Association Chicago Metro

Board (current), Grow Greater Englewood (current), and Blacks in Green (current). She also currently is inaugural Equity Visiting Scholar at Feeding America. Dr. Odoms-Young received her B.S. in foods and nutrition from the University of Illinois Urbana-Champaign and M.S./Ph.D. in community nutrition from Cornell University. Additionally, she completed a family research consortium postdoctoral fellowship examining family processes in diverse populations at the The Pennsylvania State University and the University of Illinois Urbana-Champaign, as well as a community health scholars fellowship in community-based participatory research at the University of Michigan School of Public Health.

Haley Oliver, Ph.D., is 150th Anniversary professor and assistant dean for online programs in the College of Agriculture, and the director of the U.S. Agency for International Development (USAID) Feed the Future Food Safety Innovation Lab. As director of the Food Safety Innovation Lab, she develops and oversees USAID's food safety research portfolio currently implemented in Senegal, Kenya, Bangladesh, Cambodia, Nigeria, and Nepal. She has more than 10 years of food security field experience in low- and middle-income economies. Dr. Oliver's domestic research focuses on foodborne pathogens in emerging food systems (e.g., cellular agriculture) with an emphasis on practical and feasible control strategies. Throughout her tenure, she has taught food microbiology, food safety, sanitation, and related subjects. She is deeply committed to active learning and has worked tirelessly to ensure diversity, equity, and inclusion in her classroom and research programs. Dr. Oliver has received the U.S. Department of Agriculture (USDA) and the Association of Public and Land-Grant Universities John Morrill Award, Purdue University Carine Alexander Spirit of the Land-Grant Award, USDA Food and Agriculture Science Excellence in Teaching Regional Career Award, Charles B. Murphy Teaching Award, and International Association for Food Protection James M. Jay Diversity in Food Award. She completed her B.S. in molecular biology and microbiology at the University of Wyoming and received her Ph.D. in food science, with minors in epidemiology and microbiology, at Cornell University.

Christian Peters, Ph.D., M.S., is research leader of the U.S. Department of Agriculture (USDA) Agricultural Research Service (ARS) Food Systems Research Unit in Burlington, Vermont. He came to USDA in 2021 to establish this new unit, the first at ARS to focus on food systems. Dr. Peters studies the sustainability of food systems using computational modeling and interdisciplinary research. Some of his best-known work includes the development of a modeling framework for estimating land requirements of diets and human carrying capacity and an approach for mapping potential foodsheds. Before joining ARS, Dr. Peters was associate professor in the Friedman School of Nutrition Science and Policy at Tufts University, where he taught in the Agriculture, Food and Environment graduate degree program for 11 years. He joined Tufts University as assistant professor in 2010 and was promoted to associate professor, with tenure, in 2016. Dr. Peters received his B.S. in environmental sciences from Rutgers, The State University of New Jersey, and his M.S. and Ph.D. in soil and crop sciences from Cornell University.

Guy Poppy, D.Phil, CB, FmedSci, is executive chair of the Biotechnology and Biological Sciences Research Council (BBSRC) at UK Research and Innovation (UKRI) and the UKRI executive sponsor of food (including agriculture and health) research and innovation. He previously served as the Food Standard Agency's (FSA's) chief scientific adviser (CSA) from 2014 to 2020. In this role, Dr. Poppy provided expert scientific advice to the U.K. government and played a critical role in helping to understand how scientific developments would shape the work of the FSA, as well as the strategic implications of any possible changes. His series of CSA reports have reached a wide audience and have had an impact on issues ranging from antimicrobial resistance to big data and whole genome sequencing to the Food Hygiene Rating Scheme. After completing his term of 6 years at the FSA, Dr. Poppy became the program director for the UKRI's Strategic Priorities Fund (SPF) Transforming the UK Food Systems program, a £47.5 million interdisciplinary research program that brings together researchers from almost 40 research organizations and more than 200 private- and public-sector organizations, including almost 20 government departments/agencies. From July 2022 to June 2023, he was deputy executive chair of BBSRC, focused on strategy and external engagement within BBSRC and UKRI and engagement with stakeholders of the biosciences. Dr. Poppy has significant research experience in food systems and food security and has advised governments around the world on these issues. He has published more than 100 peer-reviewed papers, including a number of highly cited articles on risk assessment, analysis, and communication. He was appointed Companion of the Order of Bath (CB) in the Queen's Birthday Honours 2021 and made a fellow of the Academy of Medical Sciences in 2022. Dr. Poppy holds a B.Sc. in biology from Imperial College London and a D.Phil in chemical ecology from Oxford University.

Sharon Ross, Ph.D., M.P.H., is program director in the Nutritional Science Research Group, Division of Cancer Prevention, National Cancer Institute (NCI), National Institutes of Health. In this capacity, she is responsible for directing, coordinating, and managing a multidisciplinary research grant portfolio in diet, nutrition, and cancer prevention. Prior to joining NCI, Dr. Ross worked at the Center for Food Safety and Applied Nutrition, Food and

Drug Administration (FDA). At FDA, she was involved in scientific review and regulation development for health claim labeling. Before FDA, Dr. Ross was a cancer prevention fellow in the Division of Cancer Prevention and Control, NCI. Dr. Ross holds a B.S. in nutrition and dietetics from the University of New Hampshire; an M.S. in nutritional sciences from the University of Connecticut; an M.P.H. from Johns Hopkins University School of Public Health with an emphasis in epidemiology; and a Ph.D. in nutritional sciences from the University of Maryland, College Park. She did her doctoral dissertation research in the Laboratory of Cellular Carcinogenesis and Tumor Promotion at NCI, where her research topic concerned the effects of retinoids in growth, differentiation, and cell adhesion.

Sylvia Rowe, M.A.T., is president of SR Strategy, which addresses the science–communications–policy continuum on a broad range of global food system issues, including agriculture, food, nutrition, and sustainability. She is also adjunct professor at the University of Massachusetts Amherst and Tufts Friedman School of Nutrition Science and Policy. Ms. Rowe is a member of the National Academies of Sciences, Engineering, and Medicine Food and Nutrition Board and the Roundtable on Obesity Solutions, and served as chair of the Food Forum from 2015 to 2021. She served as a committee member for the National Academies report Communicating Science Effectively: A Research Agenda. Ms. Rowe is contributing editor and columnist of *Nutrition Today*, serves on the Tuft's Nutrition Advisory Council, and has been recognized as an Honorary Member of the Academy of Nutrition and Dietetics (AND). Previously, Ms. Rowe served as president and chief executive officer of the International Food Information Council (IFIC) and IFIC Foundation in Washington, DC. She has served on several boards and advisory committees of the following: American Heart Association; The Obesity Society; Food Allergy and Anaphylaxis Network; American Society for Nutrition; Washington DC. Mayor's Commission on Food, Nutrition and Health; Grains for Health Foundation; University of Rochester Medical Center; Food and Drug Law Institute; Society for Nutrition Education Foundation; Maryland Title IX Commission; and the American Society of Association Executives Foundation. She is also a member of the International Women's Leadership Forum, the National Press Club, and several scientific societies. Ms. Rowe received a bachelor's degree from Wellesley College and was awarded a master's degree from Harvard University, both with honors.

Pamela Starke-Reed, Ph.D., is deputy administrator for nutrition, food safety, and product quality/new uses at the U.S. Department of Agriculture (USDA) Agricultural Research Service (ARS). She also serves as ethics officer and scientific integrity officer for ARS. Prior to ARS, she served at the National Institutes of Health (NIH) as deputy director of the Division of Nutrition Research Coordination, coordinating ongoing research on nutritional sciences, obesity, and physical activity. Her previous positions include 10 years with the National Institute on Aging, NIH, as director of the Office of Nutrition and program director for the Nutrition and Metabolism and Protein Structure and Function research programs. Other previous positions include biologist with the Food and Drug Administration's Center for Food Safety and Applied Nutrition and assistant professor with the Department of Medicine of The George Washington University (GWU). Since 1991, Dr. Starke-Reed has served as adjunct professor with the GWU Medical Center in Washington, DC. She serves as co–executive secretary for the Interagency Committee for Human Nutrition Research (ICHNR) under the chairs of the undersecretary for Research, Education, and Economics, USDA, and the assistant secretary of health, U.S. Department of Health and Human Services. She earned her B.S. in biology at St. Lawrence University and her Ph.D. in pathology at Hahnemann University.

Mary T. Story, Ph.D., M.S., R.D., is professor of global health and family medicine and community health and associate director for academic programs at the Duke Global Health Institute at Duke University. Prior to starting this position in January 2014, she was senior associate dean for academic and student affairs and professor in the Division of Epidemiology and Community Health in the School of Public Health, University of Minnesota, where she was also adjunct professor in the Department of Pediatrics, School of Medicine. Since 2005, Dr. Story has directed the Robert Wood Johnson Foundation's national program Healthy Eating Research, which explores policy-relevant solutions to preventing child obesity and improving nutrition. Dr. Story's research has focused especially on youth from low-income and minority communities, and much of her research has been on American Indian reservations. She has nearly 500 scientific publications on child and adolescent nutrition and obesity. In 2010, Dr. Story was elected to the Institute of Medicine (now the National Academy of Medicine). She was co–vice chair of the National Academies of Sciences, Engineering, and Medicine Roundtable on Obesity Solutions from 2013 to 2019. She served on the 2015–2020 Dietary Guidelines Advisory Committee with the U.S. Department of Health and Human Services and the U.S. Department of Agriculture. She also served a 6-year term on the National Academies Food and Nutrition Board. Dr. Story holds an M.S. in food science from the University of Tennessee and a Ph.D. in nutrition science from Florida State University. She is a registered dietitian.

Patrick J. Stover, Ph.D., is director of the Institute for Advancing Health through Agriculture and professor of biochemistry and biophysics at Texas

A&M University. The Stover research group investigates the fundamental chemical, biochemical, genetic, and epigenetic mechanisms and their associated pathways within the one-carbon metabolic network, which underlie the relationships among nutrition; metabolism; and risk for birth defects, cancer, and neurodegenerative diseases. Previously, Dr. Stover was vice chancellor and dean for agriculture and life sciences at Texas A&M AgriLife. As vice chancellor, he oversaw coordination and collaboration of the agriculture, academic, and research programs across The Texas A&M University System, as well as four state agencies: Texas A&M AgriLife Research, Texas A&M AgriLife Extension Service, Texas A&M Veterinary Medical Diagnostic Laboratory, and Texas A&M Forest Service. And as dean, Dr. Stover led more than 7,000 students and 330 faculty members in 15 academic departments. Additionally, he previously directed the Division of Nutritional Sciences at Cornell University. Dr. Stover is an elected member of the National Academy of Sciences and a fellow of the American Association for the Advancement of Science. He is also former president of the American Society for Nutrition and has served two terms on the National Academies of Sciences, Engineering, and Medicine Food and Nutrition Board. Dr. Stover received his Ph.D. in biochemistry and molecular biophysics from the Medical College of Virginia.